HUMOR
THERAPY

HUMOR THERAPY

THE ART OF SMILING FOR OTHERS

DAVID MANN

iUniverse®

HUMOR THERAPY
THE ART OF SMILING FOR OTHERS

iUniverse books may be ordered through booksellers or by contacting:

iUniverse
1663 Liberty Drive
Bloomington, IN 47403
www.iuniverse.com
1-800-Authors (1-800-288-4677)

ISBN: 978-1-4917-6142-7 (sc)
ISBN: 978-1-4917-6144-1 (hc)
ISBN: 978-1-4917-6143-4 (e)

Print information available on the last page.

iUniverse rev. date: 03/09/2015

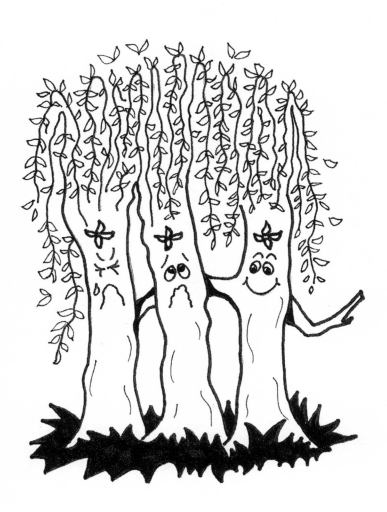

Daniel Hammond was a beautiful spirit that
was taken from earth too soon.
His loving attitude and compassion for others has
inspired me to live life to the max in his honor.
Daniel's smooth humor was clever, profound, and always on time.
He was a wise old man in a teenage body and will
be remembered by friends and family forever.
In the Land of Rihm, an imaginary place,
we will forever laugh together.

In Daniel's own words:

*The land of Rihm is a place that cannot be
gotten to by trying to get there.
You must first forget that you are trying to get
there, and then just end up there.
It's all quite simple if you know how to do it.
Now you're asking yourself, "How can I forget
that I want to go someplace?"
Well, that part is simple. You first have to
find the Land of Forgetfulness.
If you are lucky and come out on the right side of
the Land of Forgetfulness, you'll be in Rihm.
The reason that I know all these things is that I have been there,
and now I will relate to you my journey to the Land of Rihm.*

Daniel Hammond, 1985–2004

CONTENTS

PREFACE

People can be like thermometers.
When it comes to humor, some people measure the temperature at hand and only make a subtle change based on who is near them. When others laugh, so do they. When no one is laughing, they remain quiet. Just like thermometers, they only mirror the environment of those in the room.

People can be like thermostats.
When it comes to humor, some people adjust the temperature at hand, making all the difference in the world to people near them. When others laugh, so do they—but not the loudest, for they do not want to overshadow the source of the laughter. When no one is laughing, they softly create the atmosphere for laughter to grow. Just as thermostats do, they change the environment for the good of those in the room.

This book is about how I discovered how to be a humor thermostat.

My journey takes me from being a class clown to becoming a professional humor therapist. We will look at mishaps from which I learned valuable lessons, the definition of humor therapy and how to use conversation to lift spirits.

I will share my special antidotes and secret techniques that will allow you to use humor as a healing practice for loved ones in need of a laugh.

Several of my closest friends offer their perspectives, examples, and original quotes.

I have also included many types of humor questions, recipes, puns, poems, sight gags, and humor tools to try with others. I hope you find this book helpful and informative as you discover the hidden "elf" in yourself.

At any given moment, there are fellow human beings in need of a positive humor interaction. It could be a panicky mother struggling with her children in public, a stressed-out teenager in line at the grocery store, or even a stern-faced executive at the water cooler. They all need a kind word followed with a smile.

As you read this book, I hope you discover that it is quite easy to uplift others through conversational humor and purposeful humor tools.

During the last century, doctors would make house calls. They would travel through the countryside and tend to the sick. They didn't know exactly what medical instruments they would need for each trip, so they would gather all the basic tools into their doctor's bag and set off to heal their neighbors.

In this book, I describe an imaginary doctor's bag filled with humor tools for you to carry with you at all times. As you travel toward others in need of a smile, remember to use only what you need. Your personality and compassionate bedside manner are the most important tools you will ever need.

ACKNOWLEDGMENTS

Many thanks to all the contributors who shared their
comments and thoughts included in this book.
Special thanks to the following friends who helped
with proofreading, editing, grammar corrections,
and humor support prior to publishing:
Melanie Wilbur
Crystal Emerick
David Dennis
Sandi Smith

And, most of all, thanks to Debbie Mann for illustrations
and inspiration for a project that took way too long.

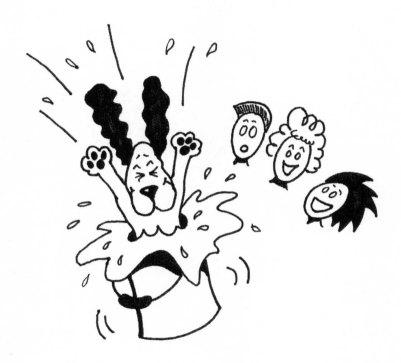

Humor is a gift best shared with friends who
share a common longing for zest and zeal.

Chapter 1

MY STORY AND MANY LESSONS LEARNED

So how exactly does someone acquire the skills of professional humor therapy? Where does it start? For me, a love of humor started out in the most common way—by being a great class clown. I can't say that my early dealings with humor were therapeutic, but they did instill a love of humor that cultivated the skills I now use for healing others with humor. This greater understanding of the power of humor also allowed me to touch hearts in new ways without leaving victims along the way. But keep in mind that it took me a while to get to that point, and I made a lot of mistakes along the way.

My appreciation for humor began during my high school years. It seemed to be the only way for me to get validation and attention from my classmates. I quickly learned that zany behavior and unpredictable actions prompted great support from my circle of friends. I really loved the praise and attention after a great humorous moment.

My most common technique was the "pie scream" which sounded like *pa-high* with a strong accent on the *high* sound. I would simply shout out this high-pitched sound in quiet situations such as the cafeteria, hallway, assembly gatherings, and sometimes during basketball games. The key was to make it loud yet discreet so heads would turn and people would look around to see where the odd sound had originated. Shock value added to my friends' laughter as heads would turn. At first only my closest peers knew it was me. After a couple of months, this low-key prank grew into a beast as I increasingly got requests to do it in serious settings such as class lectures, restaurants, and outside the principal's office. Unfortunately, I grew into a puppet that responded to these requests like a pull-string doll. As I look back now, I was being used. But I truly loved the praise and pats on the back as my reputation grew as *the funny guy* and *crazy Dave*. During my senior year of high school, I decreased the number of *pie* outbursts and only did it on special occasions to impress the ladies. For some reason, I felt as if it demonstrated rebelliousness, which was a desirable high school trait.

During this phase, I adapted another technique called the *sign smacker*.

While walking along a street sidewalk, I would calculate about twenty feet from a metal street sign. Then, bolting toward the sign, I would continually look back at my friends to make it appear that I was focused on them and not the sign. The trick was to create shock among as many onlookers as possible. With great timing and precise steps, I would raise my hand just over my ear and slap the side of the stop sign hard as I fell backward onto the sidewalk. (Stop signs made the best sound due to their size, shape, and floppiness.) Most observers would see the peripheral vision of running, hear a loud smack, and they would focus on the fall. Everyone in my group would laugh as I bounced up and quickly joined them. We walked briskly to remove ourselves from the scene, all the while evaluating the shocked faces of anyone who had caught a glance of the incident.

As I look back on it, this was a very bad version of crying wolf and collecting laughs at the expense of others. I can only imagine the thoughts of onlookers who would shake their heads in disapproval, as my group would keep laughing until they were out of sight. The only true lesson learned for me was that incongruent humor works, though I started to feel bad for the observing victims left behind. The unexpected slapstick comedy I was developing was later refined into softer techniques. This way I could continue my humorous ways without the negative impressions left behind.

Next, I redirected my attention to pranks on individuals. I enjoyed these funny antics, because the only victims were teachers. My choir class was the best environment, because it allowed me to pull something off without anyone knowing I was really the one engineering the prank. One time, sitting in the auditorium during choir class with forty classmates around me, I waited for the precise moment when the teacher was not looking. I lowered myself to the floor and crawled under the seats toward the back of the auditorium. I lit an incense cone, placed it on the cement floor (fire safety first), and crawled back to my seat and waited, all the while getting quiet snickers from classmates who had witnessed my efforts. Unfortunately, the teacher smelled the incense and called for a fire evacuation of the auditorium. I don't believe she had ever smelled incense before and she only focused on the smell of something burning. I shivered at the possibility that someone would turn me in to be expelled from school. I was lucky, and my cover was not blown. Hours later, I received encouraging praise and many accolades.

After getting away with this, I quickly started to plan the next funny stunt. Each week in choir class a student would present a musical show-and-tell moment. I could barely sing and had no musical instrument talents; I would get very annoyed with some of my classmates as they performed great musical scores and vocal presentations. As I look back, I was truly jealous of their talents. I took advantage of the fact that our teacher did not know our skills beforehand, so with the support of my peers, I volunteered to play the piano in front of the class. I walked to the front, sat confidently at the piano, opened my sheet music, and began to play. The sheet music I was playing from was "Love Story." I had to be careful that the teacher did not see the song title, because I was going to play nonsense stuff that made no sense. All was going according to plan as I played a few notes here and there, paused, and played a few keys with rhythm (I did have a musical beat in my head); I even lifted my hands into the air in between certain notes to demonstrate my fake professionalism. I was quite proud of my performance until the teacher walked over to the piano and turned the sheet music over to reveal the "Love Story" cover. The gig was up, and I politely smiled at her and returned to my seat. The audience was explosive in laughter, and my reputation was reinforced as the master prankster. The teacher was slightly annoyed yet restrained. I told myself that she thought it was funny but could not show it in front of the class. I'll never really know.

During the next choir class show-and-tell I raised the bar. As before, the teacher did not know our talents until they were demonstrated. This time, I practiced on the harmonica for one week prior, working up to playing "Kumbaya" with ease. I confidently walked to the front of the class, knowing that the teacher was watching my every move. Her dagger eyes let me know that I would not get away with another prank. I was slightly grinning as I showed her my harmonica and positioned myself. I began playing as seriously and confidently as I could. I must admit I wasn't too bad. But my harmonica playing was no match for the students who had performed prior to me with their classical scores and multitalented musical abilities. That was fine because my plan was unfolding. About forty-five seconds into my "Kumbaya," while the teacher was looking at the class, I slipped the entire harmonica into my mouth and started to breathe in and out like it was stuck. The concerned teacher quickly assisted me to the door and told me to walk quickly to the principal's office for medical attention. His office was only a couple of doors down. In the hallway, after I exited the auditorium, I removed the harmonica from my mouth and headed toward his office. Once there, I told him the whole story and apologized for putting the teacher in a panic mode. With my puppy-dog eyes, I played it off as a funny prank gone too far. I knew the entire class would never know of my apology and would again think of me as a master prankster. I was building on my reputation. The principal smiled and told me to forget about it and to return to class and tell the teacher I was fine. This prank got me laughs after the event, and I coasted on it for a couple of weeks. The power of "Did you hear what David did?" brought me a sense of accomplishment I totally enjoyed.

By this time, I was getting a little too bold and took my pranks to other classrooms. In Latin class, while the teacher was writing on the blackboard, I threw a handful of uncooked popcorn kernels into the electric fan that was on a stand in front of the class. The sound of these small projectiles flying throughout the classroom in all directions made me laugh like crazy in my head, but I remained calm as I looked at the rest of the class to see who would do such a thing. Class was disrupted and the teacher lost it. She turned red and gave the class a real verbal lashing. I remember watching the blood vessels pop out of her neck as her blood pressure was reaching the ceiling. I played it cool, and again nobody turned me in. This one was pure zany and a bit dare-devilish, but I survived it and brushed it off as another notch on my humor belt.

Finally, I went too far. I was in sociology class with a teacher we all disliked. He acted superior in his demeanor and frequently talked down to us. Wrong answers in his class were usually followed by a put-down. Several of my classmates prompted me to do something to him. I was bold, but knew if I did a prank in any form and got caught I would be in big trouble. After some resistance due to fear, I promised that I'd think of something by the following week, and I did. That weekend I heard a cute joke. It was short, nonthreatening, and straight from the brain of a grade-schooler. I even tried it out on a few friends back home to make sure it was truly funny and not over the line. I was confident. I had the perfect prank. Even if it touched a nerve, I could play it off as innocent, immature word play. I could even apologize for it if it was not received well.

During a slow period of the class when students could ask casual questions about anything in general, I asked, "Sir, have you heard that new song on the radio called 'Muddy Water Boogie'?" The teacher looked at me with a serious stare and hesitantly replied, "No." I then said with a big smile, "Well, just shake your head and you'll hear it!" Several classmates looked for a response from the teacher, knowing that if they laughed out loud, they too would be in trouble. A moment passed and he simply told me to leave his class and report to the principal's office. I was shocked. He was overreacting and I could tell he was mad. To this day, I do not remember what was in his scolding speech that followed, but I do recall feeling bad that I had crossed the line. This time, a simple apology would not repair the damage. I was in big trouble that later resulted in a suspension from his class. I learned valuable lessons that day about knowing your audience prior to making anyone in it the victim of your joke and about the power of consequences.

Boy, oh boy. I now was honored with the title of being a true class clown with guts, and my small circle of friends grew. Unfortunately, this only reminded me of that puppet called *crazy Dave* who responded to immature requests like a pull-string doll. I did not like the reputation I was developing, so I politely avoided being available for pranks and disruptive behavior. I calculated that getting kicked out of class had made me enough of a bad boy that I could coast for the rest of my senior year. So that's what I did. I played it cool—with the exception of one small prankish moment. I mention it now only to show that I still had it in me. I was still—a little bit—the amazing crazy Dave.

We were gathered in the auditorium to receive our diplomas. Each of us was called to the stage to receive the well-deserved parchment paper that proved we had passed the minimum requirements put forth by the local county education board. Everyone asked, "What is David going to do? Drop his pants? Is his hat going to explode? What is he wearing under his gown?" Well, I must admit, I teased that I would do something. I did have a reputation to uphold. But as I said before, it was just a small prankish moment. I walked across the stage, received my diploma, passed the big shots dressed in suits, paused before exiting the stage, and let out a simple but loud "*Pie!*" Many applauded and most just snickered.

That concluded my high school era of developing a sense of humor through hard lessons. It would be years before I would learn that having no victims at all makes for better laughs. By this time in my life, I had also grown tired of trying to be serious only to be discounted with "Oh really? We just thought you were joking." As a class clown, when I would try to be thoughtful or sincere, no one would take me seriously. Often, they would question my intent.

In high school I sought friends who could fill empty voids in my life, but I disregarded the simple fact that they were using me to live vicariously. Looking back, I wonder who the victim really was.

Being a class clown during my teen years helped me understand the art of the punch line, comedic timing, and what my limits were as a prankster. But while working as a traveling camp director for West Virginia University Extension Service in my early twenties, I began to understand the next level of humor, the kind of humor that heals. We were called VCAs (Volunteer Camp Assistants), a group of professional counselors that traveled throughout West Virginia during the summer to promote camp programming. At each local 4-H county camp we shared songs, games, skits, general camp knowledge, and age-appropriate fun. With this group, I learned that humor is a gift best shared with friends who share a common longing for zest in life. This job also helped me grasp the concept of camper centeredness and using humor only to help campers smile.

Class clowns, extroverts, and musically-talented staff were the most requested VCAs from each county office. About 30 percent of our staff fit this description. Being a class clown, I fit comfortably in that category. The remaining 70 percent were amazing babysitter types, experienced role models who understood youth development. They were nurturing and compassionate and knew how to interact with children. I also found this group more experienced in their love of camping and in understanding the nature of the human heart. I, along with other extroverts, could jump to the call to be the center of attention at the drop of a hat. I could lead a song or tell a joke that would bring the house down, but I envied the staff members who could talk of life-changing moments with the campers. I could surely entertain campers, but I could not touch their hearts in a meaningful way.

Spending more and more time with the 70 percent group, I realized I had much to learn about the power of humor. The next step in humor mechanics was discovering how to use humor as the mortar and not the bricks. A stand-alone joke in its simplest form is but a brick. It needs mortar to give it purpose, stability, and shape.

As I look back, there were countless times when I made a fool of myself, took center stage with sight gags, and performed comic one-man skits. The outcomes were rarely evaluated, and the clown status was hard to change. Something was missing. There were only a handful of times when friends would talk me through my mistakes to help me understand that the magic of humor was in the outcome, when someone would be uplifted.

Months later, the biggest compliment came from other camp staff members who noticed I was slowly developing heart-touching skills and using humor to comfort campers. My class clown antics were secondary as I focused on how to lift spirits and self-esteem. When someone requested me to make him or her laugh, I would hesitate, tell a soft positive joke, and fade away. When people asked me to make them feel better, I would spend time with them and help them discover laughter. I anchored my humor strategies in healing others and not in the short-term goal of getting the laugh. This new agenda left many scratching their heads and wondering, *What's with crazy Dave?* Doesn't all humor make us feel better? Yes, it does—but I wanted to be more than a joke teller. I wanted to be a healer of sorts and comfort the miserable. This is where I took the path toward being a humor professional and putting others' feelings first.

This work environment and the amazing counselors contributed to one of the biggest turning points for me. I discovered that humor is hidden in conversation. As a young VCA, I noticed that there were popular campers as well as campers who needed a little nudge in developing their social skills.

Often when I would take our cabin to the waterfront, I would notice one or two campers who would sit on the sidelines and not participate in swimming activities. I suspected that there was a reason for this, but I did not focus on getting them into the water as other counselors did. To focus on the problem was short-term, and it usually led to well-rehearsed excuses or apologies. Instead, I would sit beside them and explore their humor. Laughing at the silly side of life and talking about something like the weirdest food ever eaten created a poolside atmosphere of acceptance and laughing. Other counselors would ask, "How come you didn't get them in the water?" I would state, "We did, in our minds, and we also increased our humor IQ through joke analysis!" The poolside connection with these campers built trust and comfort that allowed them, by week's end, to ask if I would assist them into the shallow end of the pool. The humor connection was the goal, and the participation in swim activities was the by-product. It worked most of the time, but even if it didn't, I helped a lot of non-swimmers feel comfortable sitting on the sidelines enjoying the view, the atmosphere, and the sun—all the while laughing at life.

Rubbing of elbows was a technique to open a campfire in a positive fun manner, something I had learned in my twenties while sitting around the campfire at 4-H camps.

It was one of the camp's "Laws of the council circle" and described as the Native American's gift to remember that laughter was good medicine. While sitting around the campfire, all would lightly rub elbows with the person on either side of them. One hundred percent of the time, a slow spread of smiles to laughter would ensue as the elbow rubbing continued. It always ended with the campers being more attentive, focused, and relaxed before continuing on with the evening's campfire program. I use this technique to this day to warm up workshop participants and keynote audiences. I believe that starting any program with light humor leads to better outcomes.

Some of my best humor lessons came to life while gazing into those campfire flames and listening to the great storytellers.

One story told around the campfire was about finding a dead mule in the bathtub. I can't recall the full plot of the story, but I do remember that it took twenty minutes to tell. The laughs came from reenacting and pantomiming the act of carrying the mule all around town and up some stairs in a *Dumb and Dumber* manner. The punch line came when a simple question was presented at the end of the story, questioning the mule carrying effort. The response that captured most of the laughs was "No silly, what do you think I am—*stupid*?" After twenty minutes of silly motions, current catch phrases of the day, and funny faces, the crowd already thought we were pretty stupid. Hence the incongruent punch line that nobody expected. The true art of the story was to entertain the campers with creative imagery and slapstick walks (we were carrying a dead mule, you see). The prolonged story was a classic and was requested each year. There was something about the story that was familiar, traditional, and comfortable in the retelling of it. Each year the story was fresh, new, and updated. The changes to the story were subtle and sometimes built on the previous year in a passing remark like "Hey, this ain't last year, stick to the script." With a wink and a smile, the players were reminding us of the art of storytelling. The rich oral history was filled with unforgettable humor and was knee-slapping funny even when you knew the punch line.

Everyone knew the best conversational laughs would be at the breakfast table the morning after as each camper had his or her interpretation and opinion of what made the mule story funny. This was more than a joke or skit; it was a tradition of humor storytelling that connected us to a simpler time when even a silent pause with one raised eyebrow could get the best laughs. No, this was not a bust your gut, laugh-out-loud span of twenty minutes, but for many it was a profoundly deep, cathartic opportunity to relive a bit of history and feel good about yourself until next year. We looked forward to hearing it year after year. You could say that it was prescribed healing humor from the storytellers, like humor therapy.

Then I relapsed, oh so badly. I know now I had more lessons to learn.

As a camp director at a summer seasonal camp, I often took time to walk to the theater building to watch young campers practice for the talent show on the last night. A particularly hippieish counselor was assisting and directing the group of young females in the reenactment of *The Giving Tree,* a children's story of a tree that gave its all. The counselor was truly a back-to-nature type and never shaved her armpits. While standing in the back of the seating section, my assistant director and I watched the rehearsal unfold. Between the two of us, we came up with a variety of sound effects, insulting comments, and just downright disrespectful humor. Nobody heard our comments from the stage, but our jokes and sharp tongues got the best of us as we slowly laughed louder and louder—to the point that one loud laugh was too much. I think it was when the counselor raised her arms into the air showing her armpits and pretended to be a tree while the campers skipped around her. "Is she playing a tree or a bush?" was the showstopper between us. The campers and the counselor all stopped the rehearsal and looked at us. They surely did not hear us, did they? Maybe only our laughter was heard. Oh no!

We apologized and exited the building, all the while snickering and feeling we were the best humorists ever. At dinner that night, the counselor approached me and stated that the girls thought that we were laughing at their performance, and it hurt their feelings. I assured her that it was not their performance but an inside joke, and she was right that it was disrespectful to laugh inappropriately in their midst. I told her that I'd make it right with an apology.

After breakfast the following morning, I gathered all the campers outside and presented them with a formal apology. Standing beside the assistant director in front of a table with all sorts of food items, I started my speech with the facts. A cruel and heartless act had occurred the day before and we were there to set things right. With each spoken line, the assistant director and I took turns pouring, rubbing, and smearing a food item into each other's head and shoulders. It went something like this: *"Lettuce" try to make things right; we want to "catsup" to where we were before; we thought about the damage we did yesterday and "mustarded" up the strength to apologize; it was "eggs-actly" the right thing to do; you can't "beet" true friendships (canned beets); we feel like "mill worms" (oatmeal) by hurting others' feelings; we "relish" the thought of getting back to the way things were.* We looked for flowers to give to our performers but could only come up with flour (which covered our heads). We smeared each food item onto our faces and shared a camp-wide apology that was memorable and funny. The counselor thanked us, and said that it was just what her girls needed.

A few lessons were learned here: 1) humor can hurt if the receiver does not understand the source of the laughter, 2) he or she usually internalizes it and thinks less of himself or herself being the target of others' humor, and 3) most of all, the best lesson was if you break it, fix it. We were lucky enough that day to realize that a miracle was needed to repair the damage we had done. Through humor we healed, but the fact remains—we should never have created the problem. To this day, I think before I speak, and I'm always mindful of how my body language, tone, and humor may come across to others. To laugh *at* someone truly causes damage to his or her self-esteem and confidence. To laugh *with* someone truly causes growth to his or her self-esteem and confidence.

I continued to learn the dangers of humor and the misuse of pranks. There was a camp that had a tradition of giving a "spirit stick" to the best group on the last night of camp. The entire camp was divided into four tribes that competed in sports, spirit, and good sportsmanship each week. The spirit stick was handed off throughout the week for notable successes, sometimes after a lunch, and sometimes after a field day meet. The stick became the trophy and all the campers wanted to at least carry it for a few hours each day. As a final reward, the stick went home with the winning tribe leader at the end of the camp session.

This one particular week, I noticed that the groups were becoming slightly negative in their demeanor and were a bit rude after winning the stick. By the end of the week, one group was marginally ahead in all points and demonstrated bad behavior to the rest of the camp.

In an attempt to play a good humor prank on them and teach a well-deserved lesson, I borrowed the spirit stick during lunch one day and made a replica. It looked so close to the original that you really had to look closely to tell the difference. The feathers, the leather binding around the top, and even the paint job were perfect. I hid it until closing campfire. As the traditional rituals unfolded with special recognitions and honors announced, I finally retrieved the stick from the group that had been holding it all afternoon. My announcement of the winner for the week was timed just right. I laid the stick behind my seat beside the fake spirit stick and continued to tell a campfire story. At the end of the story, I picked up the fake stick and told the entire camp that spirit had not been taken to the highest level and that no one deserved the stick. I then laid the stick on the center of the campfire allowing it to burn. With a smile on my face that I thought all would notice, I stepped back as the stick began to flame. I really thought I had gotten them with a dose of "Ha, take that!" Within five seconds of placing it on the fire, at least a dozen campers bolted toward the fire to save the stick. Oh my goodness, a disaster was just about to happen! Many were about to be burned trying to save a fake spirit stick! I shouted at the top of my lungs, "Stop, I was only joking! It's a fake!" Inches from the flame, four young campers stopped and looked up at me. Nobody was laughing, and the entire camp was giving me dagger-eye stares, all the while thinking what a jerk I was. I don't remember what else was said from that point on. I just know I backpedaled enough to save face and continue on with the ending songs and campfire closing.

As we walked toward the cabins to retire, several adults approached me and asked, "What were you thinking?"

I replied, "I wish you could have seen it all play out in my mind prior to doing it. It was a hoot!"

But in reality, what a disaster! You would think that such a risk management error would have taught me better, but no—it did not. Somehow, I recuperated from this and planned another prank the following week. (When was I ever going to learn that pranks are never good?)

This one had no risk of campers jumping into the fire, just shocking the daylights out of them.

As the camp director, I sat at the apex of the circle and often fed the fire with additional sticks to keep the flame going. Nobody paid me any mind, as long as I was respectful of the skit or talent demonstration going on. I had just purchased a fake hand that looked real. With the shadows of the night dancing nearby and the campfire aglow, I picked up a small hatchet and a large piece of wood, pretending to chip it a bit while walking toward the fire. I intentionally tripped, throwing the wood to the left, the fake hand to the right, and keeping my real hand just inside my long-sleeved shirt. The hatchet appeared to have landed on my left wrist and I screamed, "Ouch!" With a loud laugh, my real hand magically grew from my shirtsleeve as I jumped up to show that it all was a big joke. From the laughter I knew I had pulled it off with no psychological damage to anyone. My timing had been perfect, and the whole incident was over within a matter of seconds. Somehow I knew that this was the best showstopper I had ever performed, and the rave reviews would classify me as the best *gotcha* artist around. I do remember that the entire group laughed. I played that moment over and over in my head as we walked to the cabins that night.

Shortly after, I was approached by a small group of adult volunteers who explained what had happened from their perspective. The moment that I faked the hand removal, a small female camper, age eight, wet her pants and began to cry. The adults quickly rushed her away from the campfire and soothed her, telling her over and over again that it was just a silly prank. Later that night, I apologized to the camper, but it was too little too late. I was no hero in her mind. The next morning, other counselors ribbed me and even thanked me for the "best one ever!" but I let each person know that I was not proud of my actions and regretted hurting such a beautiful young camper. I think this is what it took for me to realize that humor can hurt. All pranks have victims, and things that are hilarious in my mind are not as funny in the real world.

It was weeks before I tried to pull anything funny in the presence of campers. I do recall hanging a long strip of toilet tissue from my back pocket and walking through the dining hall from the rest room. I think it was then that I discovered that making *myself* the butt of jokes works best. Who knew?

Youth camping is a world where silliness and being zany can instantly capture the attention of young growing minds in a positive way. The secret is to keep reminding yourself that being a role model means that every word out of your mouth and action displayed should be for the good of others, expecting it to be seen and overheard by all. You can share humor in a variety of ways, but it's your core values that allow it to be meaningful.

One summer, I discovered hats. I filled a duffle bag full of novelty hats and occupational head attire. With each hat, I simply played myself. There were no funny voices, no characters, and no offensive puns. The surprise of pulling out a new hat during field day was a hit by itself. If a dispute emerged, a policeman hat would appear followed by smiles. If a ball was overshot in the field, I put on my jogger's headband and bolted. If there was something that happened on the field that got a laugh from other campers, a jester's hat complimented the situation. Humor was about working the funny bone while being a great role model. The campers' parents validated this with their supportive comments and applause. My laughter and positive humor was contagious. I was slowly getting it.

At one camp, I remember oversleeping the first morning. At breakfast, the older campers awarded me with a large clock made out of a tin pie plate and construction paper to wear all day.

It was their way of telling me through humor to "be on time or else."

I complied just to get smiles from the younger campers, but I could tell that it was going to be a difficult week. I had gotten off on the wrong foot, and from that point on, my style of humor and silliness did not go over well with the teens, counselors, or adult support staff.

My communication style was lacking and I needed a new strategy.

I adopted the *If you can't beat them, join them* strategy, hoping it would minimize criticism.

That week I volunteered to get water thrown in my face, pudding on my head, flour on my cheeks, and a variety of dining hall food down my back. I used a lot of slapstick humor. I always smiled and calmly remained the victim of their pranks. After all, they were having fun with it, and it was for the kids.

I wore the same shirt two days in a row (my excuse was that it was my favorite) and the next morning my entire wardrobe was on each camper. They all said that they liked my favorites, too. My shirts and shorts were all being worn by everybody standing in line at the flagpole. This prank was cleverly initiated by the adult staff as another power play. It proved that I could take a joke, but inside I hated the thought of doing all that laundry.

I realized I was losing the respect of the adults who regarded me as a clown, so I paused to reinvent myself. I knew there was more to learn to be a humorist, funny guy, comedian—or whatever I was becoming. By week's end, the campers thought I was pretty funny, but the adults were rolling their eyes and shaking their heads. One leader, under her breath, stated, "Good riddance" during departure. I survived that camp, but left feeling ineffective with my humor style.

The last few weeks that summer I focused on music and storytelling, mastering many camp songs on the guitar and perfecting several heart-touching stories for children. *Talent over humor* became my new mantra. The camping season ended on a high note and I felt energized with confidence. The sunsets, campfires, group singing, and watching children smile affected me in a profound way.

A fire within me had been kindled, and I knew that someday I would return to camping.

I spent the next few years sliding into the real workforce in a Board of Education educational supplies delivery position, as a state park lifeguard, and other "adult" jobs. They were never as great as camping, but those jobs paid better and allowed me to purchase vehicles, go on dates, and eat a better class of food.

Different work environments also allowed for new insights into my humor style. Another powerful lesson presented itself to me from an eight-year-old. This time it was more profound, and I credit it as the catalyst that changed my life in a monumental way.

While working at a state park swimming pool, I met all types of people from around the world. Proud of being personable, I was very comfortable in sharing a smile and a little humor as guests waited in line to pay and enter the changing rooms. Some of the other lifeguards would try to be funny with sharp comments and bad jokes. I thought I was the true soft humor expert, using common conversational humor with them. It was easy to just be myself and make lighthearted suggestions about how to enjoy the water and sunbathing areas. I thought I was the master until one day an eight-year-old came bouncing in half dancing and half silly-walking. He skipped a bit, spinning around, and then approaching the counter to pay. I noticed his mother still outside attending to his siblings. With a big smile, I asked the cutting-edge question, "What's up with the dancing type of walk—you got six toes?" To my surprise, the young gentleman looked up at me and responded, "No, but I only have four toes on this foot!" With a giant smile, he explained how he had lost one of his toes. I heard none of his explanation and positive story. All I could think of was, "Oh my gosh, I've said the wrong thing and how stupid of me!"

He continued talking, laughing at himself and dancing away into the dressing room. He intentionally smoothed over my blundering comment with a forgiving smile, positive attitude, and compassionate perspective. Through his laughter, he made me feel better. To this day, I suspect that he knew he was helping me learn about disabilities and how he was okay with himself. I learned so much about humor therapy that day. He smiled for me, hence my favorite saying: "Smile for others!"

Years later, after receiving a master's degree in therapeutic recreation, becoming a (CTRS) Certified Therapeutic Recreation Specialist and a (CLL) Certified Laughter Leader I worked at one of Paul Newman's Hole In The Wall therapeutic camps for seriously ill children as vice president of medical services. This gave me a better medical and therapeutic mind-set on healing and helping others. It was the turning point of my life. This was the moment I created a therapeutic imaginary doctor's bag for myself and confidently sought out those who needed a smile.

I'm currently the camp director at Camp Boggy Creek (now a Paul Newman Serious Fun facility) where I oversee camp programming. In this particular setting, humor is the best medicine and campers are the experts. They truly know how to smile, giggle, and laugh with every passing moment of their day. Their compassion for each other is amazing, and they share humor through even the most difficult struggles of daily medical routines. Each day I learn more about healing humor and the positive effects of conversational humor. My heart is forever tied to the program staff and cabin counselors who give up their summers to play and laugh with special needs youth.

Try This:

Put fifteen small items (cotton balls, bits of fabric, candy wrappers, and so forth) in your left pocket. Throughout the day, transfer one item from the left pocket to the right pocket every time you are responsible for putting a smile on another's face. Smiling at someone and receiving a smile in return counts. If you are really into this, try it for a few days. You will be surprised how focused and intentional your humor is and how it rubs off on others. I dare say this one single experiment will change your life.

You will also be pleased that you have exponentially spread goodwill and positive feelings to the world!

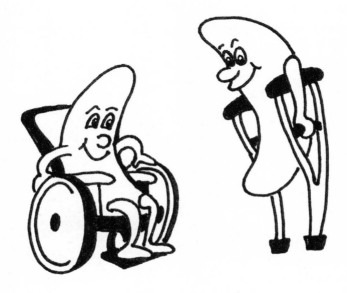

Humor therapy is like aloe. You can't spread or rub it on others without getting some of it on yourself. And, as a bonus, it heals both.

Chapter 2

WHAT IS HUMOR THERAPY?

Have you ever seen humor therapy in action? A few years ago, I watched two brothers, a nine-year-old and a seven-year-old, climbing a staircase leading to a high viewing platform at a family healing camp. They ran together until the younger boy stopped about three steps up and refused to go any further. The nine-year-old continued on to the top, looked back, and called to his brother.

"Keep climbing," he shouted. "It's beautiful up here."

The seven-year-old didn't move, obviously afraid to climb any higher. In a heartbeat, his older brother ran down to his side, leaned over, and whispered something in his ear. I couldn't hear what he said, but both boys broke into laughter, clasped hands, and tore up the stairway together.

I wish I knew what the older brother said, but I do know that whatever he said achieved two things. First, it promoted laughter and eased the seven-year-old's fears; secondly, it helped him forget about whatever was worrying him long enough to dart to the top.

In its simplest form, this is humor therapy initiated by the older brother. He understood what was needed, thought about it, and did something through conversation that helped. He helped his younger brother master a challenge, and they both enjoyed the end result.

As Todd and Janet explain it, it is all about lifting spirits when needed. After the loss of their son from cancer, they devoted their lives to volunteering at therapeutic camps to help others find lost laughter. In describing a humor therapy example, Todd shares this story: "One time when Bryan was in the hospital for chemo, we played a trick on the doctors and nurses. We placed spots of Play-Doh on his legs, covered them with a sheet, and pushed the nurse button. When she came in, we said he had a weird rash on his legs and asked whether she would take a look. A little worried, she pulled back the sheet. It was so funny to her that she called the doctor in. Concern all over his face, he entered the room. He laughed out loud, something that folks don't always do in pediatric oncology."

Here is what my niece, Fallon, says on keeping things fun with her sister: "One of the things I do to help Sage laugh is make funny faces, and it's not just one or two; it's whatever pops into my head, which makes a variety after a couple of days. We also like to make weird sounds at each other, also very random. (Mom doesn't seem to like it very much, though.) At least once a day Sage lets out a 'Meep!'"

"What exactly is humor therapy?" you ask. Well, I like to think of it this way:

Imagine standing on a stage and your goal is to lift the spirits and mood of an audience. You would probably use humor resources from the world of jokes, gags, or impressions to create a smile. All in all, you would entertain them from a distance in a monologue format. This example is pure humor but not necessarily therapeutic. It is one directional.

Now imagine you are given the same goal of lifting someone's spirit, but this time you must do it with only one person while seated beside him or her in the audience seating area. You would probably use conversation, interactions, or interpersonal skills to elicit a smile. This example is closer to describing humor therapy, as it requires dialogue, closer proximity, and the attempt to actually assess his or her mood while creating a smile. It is interactive and two directional.

Humor therapy in action can also be described as *simply meeting them where they are.* Or, as my mom would say, "If you don't laugh like you do at home, you should be." Ha! Okay, Mom's quote is a stretch here, but it does make you think, huh?

Let's continue with this train of thought.

The closer you are to the non-smiling, the better you are able to actually interact more effectively.

Humor therapy is prescribed and dispersed slowly, a little at a time. Offering too much can make you appear like a clown, and offering too little can be ineffective. When someone you know is feeling down, you don't start juggling or making balloon animals; you interact to help him or her discover the humor personally. If you do this correctly, the person will never know you had a hand in leading the process. Humor therapy is such an easy concept, but most people confuse it with humor, comedy, and laughter. Don't get me wrong; these are great tools for entertaining, but they are not humor therapy.

Now let's complicate things a little.

Humor therapy and therapeutic humor are often confused. What is the difference, and how can you tell which is which? Answer: the last word of the term describes what it is. It is simply *humor* or *therapy*.

In other words, therapeutic humor is uplifting humor that comes in many forms and promotes feeling better. Humor therapy is a medical model form of therapy prescribed with thoughtful, purposeful, and intentional outcomes.

Therapeutic Humor
The Association for Applied and Therapeutic Humor (www.aath.org) defines therapeutic humor as the following:

Any intervention that promotes health and wellness by stimulating a playful discovery, expression or appreciation of the absurdity or incongruity of life's situations. This intervention may enhance health or be used as a complementary treatment of illness to facilitate healing or coping, whether physical, emotional, cognitive, social or spiritual.

Therapeutic humor casts a wide net in its description. All positive, uplifting humor is therapeutic if a person is in need of it. If I'm feeling down, a good sitcom, pun, or silly joke lifts my spirits. At one time or another, most people have thought, *I just need a good laugh.* Sometimes it is a matter of redirection—simply placing yourself in a fun environment or setting aside an hour in front of a TV set with your favorite sitcom. During this escape, you may find yourself feeling slightly calmer, in a better frame of mind, and focused on the lighter side of life. Any type of positive humor will offer relief and comfort. Watching cats do silly things on the Internet can turn a bad day into a pleasant moment that forces you to forget your day-to-day miseries.

Remember: it is humor, and it makes you feel better.

Humor Therapy
The American Cancer Association (www.cancer.org) defines humor therapy as the following:

Humor therapy is the use of humor for the relief of physical pain and stress. It is used as a complementary method to promote health and cope with illness.

Whether or not you work in the medical field, you can use the tools and techniques presented in this book to help others in need. You can achieve positive outcomes by your involvement, close interactions, facilitation, guidance, assistance, and simple prescriptive measures.

Imagine you are a doctor who has been asked to heal a person's lack of humor (*humoritis*). You would assess the patient's condition, create a plan to help with his or her healing, implement the idea, and then evaluate the whole process. You can even imagine that you carry a doctor's bag filled with pleasant jokes, puns, fun stories, and silly ideas. Once you identify the issue or problem at hand, you simply provide the remedy that is needed.

Remember: it's based on a medical model that, once prescribed, can heal.

So in its simplest form:
Going to a comedy club with the guys: therapeutic humor.
Going to a comedy club with Bob because he just lost his job and the guys are intentionally trying to raise his spirits (and they have planned this outing all week): humor therapy.

Dropping off joke books to someone in the hospital: therapeutic humor.
Lifting spirits via funny conversations with someone in the hospital room: humor therapy.

Watching a marathon of your favorite sitcoms alone on a rainy day: therapeutic humor.
Watching a marathon of your favorite sitcoms with your spouse while she is sick with a stomach virus and commenting on how "life is good": humor therapy.

Putting together a Caribbean dinner party for the new neighbors: therapeutic humor.
Putting together a Caribbean dinner party for someone who is feeling down: humor therapy.

Going to the park to watch children laugh and play: therapeutic humor.
Going to the park with Bob to watch children laugh and play because he misses his daughter who is away for the summer: humor therapy.

Choosing which comic movie is best for date night with your spouse: therapeutic humor.
Choosing which comic movie is best for someone who is stressed out: humor therapy.

Laughing out loud with your best friend (trick question): therapeutic humor or humor therapy—it depends.

Notice how the definitions of therapeutic humor and humor therapy can become cloudy and overlap depending on the circumstances, intent, and usage of humor. Fear not; I look at it this way—in this day and age you can describe almost anything as therapeutic humor if it puts a smile on someone's face while humor therapy is intentional and purposeful. Humor therapy is a piece of the pie and therapeutic humor is the whole pie.

And if the whole concept of humor therapy versus therapeutic humor is still confusing, think of it this way. The first word is an adjective while the second word is a noun. Humor therapy is *therapy* and therapeutic humor is *humor*.

Let's look at the nouns.

While working in a behavior hospital I learned that art *therapy*, music *therapy*, and horticulture *therapy* were serious program options when they were presented by mental health professionals. Whether they were prescribed to enhance social skills, build better hand/eye coordination, or tap into emotions, they all assisted in the healing of patients. Art, music, and horticulture are simply adjectives of a specific *therapy*.

Therapeutic *art* can be art that pleases the eye. It includes visuals that are positive and make one feel pleasant. Therapeutic *music* can be music that relaxes me or puts me in a good mood. Therapeutic *horticulture* can be growing an avocado seed in the kitchen window. All are super activities but not true therapy unless prescribed. Shopping *therapy* is real if it's prescribed by a psychologist to help a patient deal with chrometophobia (fear of money) or enochlophobia (fear of crowds). Therapeutic *shopping* is when I have an extra twenty bucks and spend a little time at the mall seeking a T-shirt with a funny message.

The remainder of this book will deal solely with humor therapy and how to develop your own bag of tricks. Along the way you'll learn how to interact using conversational tools. So let's get started.

The APIE Model

Prescribing humor therapy is as easy as making a pie (APIE).

This acronym, from *The Dynamic Nurse-Patient Relationship* by Ida Jean in 1961, is a modified scientific method that stands for *assess, plan, implement,* and *evaluate.*

The components of the model begin with assessment and go through to the evaluation process; then it repeats when needed. Sometimes each step is brief and takes only seconds, while other steps can take months. As long as the steps of APIE are sequential, intentional, and supported with compassion, the outcome will help promote smiles and the uplifting of others.

I can sometimes thoughtfully assess and plan an intervention of humor in seconds and then implement a clever conversation that is well timed and effective. An example might be discussing my dad's pickled egg recipe. After the conversation, I will evaluate the total interaction and remind myself, *Well that worked okay, but the next time I will not go into so much detail about the pickled eggs recipe.* (Not meaning to change the subject here, but everyone should know that the recipe secret is to use the juice from pickled beets and not the juice from plain canned beets.) *Assess* the situation, *plan* on what to say next, *implement* through conversation, and, sometime later, *evaluate* how things went.

An example of APIE is my parents' Thanksgiving get-togethers. A few years ago I would visit my mom and dad for a couple of days in their isolated house in the woods. There was nothing much to do but watch TV and play board games. Every night we would pull out Scrabble or Trivial Pursuit. I tried a variety of other new board games, but my dad would have nothing to do with them. After several years of narrowing it down to these two games, I discovered something. When we played Trivial Pursuit for three hours, the conversation sometimes lingered with sidebar topics of past experiences or great memories that the Trivial Pursuit question had reminded us of. We would laugh quite a bit during these game sessions. After the game was over, we would retire for the night feeling as though we had shared a part of ourselves and connected as a family. But during the actual Scrabble game we would focus on the wooden letters, and conversation was limited. After the game was over, my parents and I would retire for the night feeling competitive and slightly unexpressed with our thoughts. We didn't share any fun stories during these evenings. So I started buying several different themed versions of Trivial Pursuit and the sidebar comic conversations continued. I *assessed* an issue of not sharing fun past experiences, came up with a *plan* to change the general feelings of the evening, *implemented* the games, and *evaluated* the whole process. My parents never knew I was doing this, but I could tell by their behavior that they were enjoying it more than ever. I was pleased with the outcome.

Here is another example of the APIE model.

My brother-in-law, Joe, got a beautiful tattoo on his shoulder that was a scene of ant-like cartoon characters playing musical instruments in front of a colorful mountain backdrop. I was impressed with his personal design. He showed it to my wife Debbie (his sister), and we swooned at the colors and original art. Then we asked what Mack and Ina (his parents) thought of it. He said that they did not know and that he was hesitant to show them because they were not happy about tattoos. I noticed that he wore shirts with sleeves to cover the tattoo up while they were around. Joe's worries about acceptance from his parents, even at his age, were quite sweet and innocent, and tugged at all of our heartstrings. The thought of sharing the news with family was a bit unnerving, to say the least. I don't remember how, but one day the word got out to Ina. It was probably from me in a passing conversation with her about family members with tattoos. She smiled and accepted it since Joe was an adult and living on his own. It did not bother her in the least, but she did ask, "You think he will ever tell us?" Debbie and I looked at each other, and then replied, "We'll help with that."

Since I had already let the cat out of the bag, I felt responsible for doing this without causing harm to Joe's trust.

So we formed a plan to assist Joe with telling Mack and Ina about his tattoo, whether he was ready or not.

A few days later, Debbie and I started pressuring Joe to just go ahead and tell his parents about the tattoo. He did not think the timing was right; he said he thought later would be better—maybe in a few weeks. We told him kiddingly that if he did not tell them, we would. He agreed to share it all with them soon.

That following weekend, Joe, Mack, Ina, Debbie, and I met at the mall's food court to enjoy a snack before parting ways to shop.

Earlier that day, Ina had put a temporary tattoo on her forearm and covered it with long sleeves. Her role in this plan was the key to the humor portion, as she was the "Aha!" lady.

So here we all were, sitting at a small table at the food court, eating and avoiding the whole tattoo issue and giving Joe the *look* as if we might say something. Ina then set the plan into motion. She looked Joe in the eye and asked, "So, Joe, anything new in your life? Have you done anything out of the norm that you might want to share with us?" Joe looked at Debbie and me thinking we had sold him out. I said, "Hey, don't look at *us!*" Joe was getting anxious and his eyes shifted back and forth to Ina, Debbie, Mack, and me.

Ina said, "Ever consider getting a tattoo like the one I got?" As she said this, she pulled up her sleeve and showed off her temporary tattoo. It looked quite real. We all broke into laughter.

Joe grinned slowly, and as his mood shifted he first giggled and then broke into relieved laughter.

The tension was gone, and Ina and Mack set the tone for him to finally pull up his own sleeve to show off his colorful tattoo artwork. For the following ten minutes, Joe confidently retold the story of how he had designed it, adding details of what each character meant to him and how he planned on enhancing it later. It was a pure pleasure sitting back and watching this whole event unfold with laughter. We had assessed, planned, and implemented the entire event. Evaluation took only seconds with Debbie saying to me, "Good job!"

Another way to implement the APIE model is allowing humor to grow on its own, nudging it along based on the situation.

For example, while on a cruise with the family, we sat at our table as the waiter came by to pick up the finished plates. In doing so, he accidentally dropped a couple of plates and silverware on the floor. The entire family laughed at the awkward moment and quickly let the waiter know we were not bothered. I could see from the expression on his face that he was expecting a negative reaction from us. Maybe that was what he was used to. We smoothed out the accident with positive comments, even adding slight humor to the event. The waiter left feeling relieved. About ten minutes later, the waiter returned to assist with an after-meal coffee. His timing was perfect. As he picked up a small saucer from the center of the table, he pretended to lose his grip on the saucer and caught it before it hit the table. He did this on purpose to add humor to the prior mishap. As he stood there smiling, we broke into another round of laughter, stating in various ways, "Good one!"

As we processed and evaluated the event later that night, it was obvious that we had assessed the situation, planned our comments carefully, and implemented humor with acceptance. This allowed the waiter the opportunity to feel better.

As a family, we prescribed what was needed to comfort the waiter about his mishap.

But wait a minute—maybe it was the *waiter* who had assessed the situation, planned a touch of added humor, faked a second mishap, and created the opportunity for *us* to feel better!

Either way, everyone involved shared in the success of the outcome.

Humor therapy can be that simple. See a need, size it up, do something to help, and rejoice in the results.

Try This:

I mentioned earlier about carrying an imaginary doctor's bag filled with jokes, puns, stories, and ideas. By doing this, you will be equipped with what you need, when you need it—for any occasion that requires the help of humor.

Fill your personalized doctor's bag with a variety of tools, such as

a funny poem that you learned as a child;
an exaggeration of what you see at the moment;
the description of how you feel before you sneeze;
a story of one of your most embarrassing moments;
a pun that feels right and is cleverly injected into normal conversation;
a well-practiced silly face that highlights a point;
an eyebrow that lifts when you want to express "Oh really?";
hand movements that exaggerate your descriptions;
questions that end silent pauses;
intentional comments that allow for questions like "What on earth are you talking about?";
sound effects that highlight a point;
patience that rubs off on others;
a description of a household object used differently or oddly;
a nursery rhyme that is changed or updated;

compassion;
listening skills that demonstrate your interest;
empathy and/or sympathy when needed;
a magic trick; and
sometimes just picking up the lunch check.

Once, while talking to a friend who had just sneezed, we discussed the various types of sneezes that were possible. There are chocolate sneezes that sound like *Hershey,* cobbler sneezes that sound like *a shoe,* bubblegum sneezes that sound like *I chew,* seamstress sneezes that sound like *I sew,* fly swatter sneezes that sound like *ah shoo,* and many more.

Fill your bag with tactics that work for you. Games, songs, favorite quotes, movie lines, and idioms are all wonderful items to have on hand.

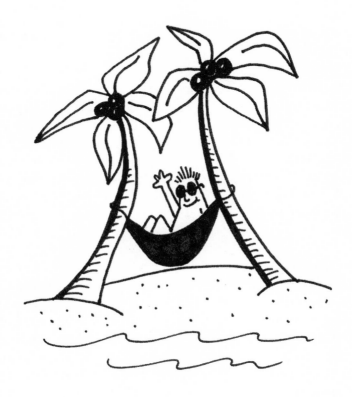

Humor therapists do not just humor others; they adjust
the environment for humor to develop on its own.

CHAPTER 3

THE ART OF CONVERSATION

After my epiphany of using humor to heal, the next step was to pursue the right credentials to go along with it.

This included getting a master's degree in therapeutic recreation, becoming a certified laughter leader, becoming a certified therapeutic recreation specialist, being a board member of the Association for Applied and Therapeutic Humor, and reviewing all the latest humor research. What exactly do I do today? How am I applying these techniques in everyday life and in my career? The answer is very simple: I promote Art Linkletter's advice when he said, "The best things happen to people who make the best of things that happen to them."

Today I believe that conversational humor in its simplest form is the best positive catalyst for helping people understand Art's quote. Art was famous for his interviewing style with children. When asked how he did it, he replied that he just brought himself down to their level and talked. Watching him converse on TV you could see him using positive, uplifting verbal interactions and cues. His warm fatherly smile and demeanor truly influenced me, as I'm sure it did millions of viewers. This was so simple, yet so powerful.

To understand the power of humor, one must accept the fact that the last couple of decades of research have shown that laughter has many benefits for the entire body. This includes improvements and increased stimulation to the respiratory system, sympathetic nervous system, immune system, muscular system, digestive system, and even to the brain. A body of work by Paul E. McGee, Ph. D. on health and humor describes psychoneuroimmunology (PNI) which is the study of the interaction between psychological processes and the nervous and immune systems of the human body. Dr. McGee has published over a dozen books along with many scientific articles on humor therapy. Discover more about his research on health and humor online at laughterremedy.com.

Today ongoing research supports that laughter and humor may have therapeutic value and makes a significant contribution to health.

Humor also fosters a positive and hopeful attitude that leads us away from feelings of depression and helplessness. It gives us a better sense of perspective about daily problems and changes our emotional response to stress. And to date, it has no negative side effects!

The science does not lie. Humor does so much good. It's a wonder the world doesn't practice it daily. Wait a minute; it *is* practiced every day by millions. I see it all the time online with *LOL*.

As a humor therapist, I often have the opportunity to help others in a variety of ways. I never walk into a room as if I'm the answer. I walk into a room and check the mood and atmosphere before I find my place. Sometimes it is as simple as providing opportunities for others to smile and forget their worries; other times it is just a matter of providing the small spark that gets things going. I pretend that I'm a humor-doctor and have my doctor's bag filled with many tools of the trade. The techniques and skills of reading body language, starting conversations, knowing jokes and funny anecdotes, having examples of life experiences, and making comments that promote smiles—all of these come in handy.

The tools I use follow a basic model, an understanding first and foremost of using the Hippocratic oath, *do no harm.* This includes knowing that positive, constructive humor raises a person's self-esteem, is supportive in nature, reduces tension, breaks down barriers, relaxes people, stimulates new ideas, and creates a positive atmosphere for all involved. Contrast this with negative, destructive humor that lowers self-esteem, belittles people, creates tension, creates barriers, creates defensiveness, closes off creative thought, and focuses on negatives in general.

The tools in my imaginary bag are infinite and ever-changing, as I prescribe just what is needed for each situation.

If you think about it, parents do this each and every day by sprinkling love and advice to their children in just the right doses. Parents nurture, guide, and coach their child's growth through any given issue or grief. They support with love and a smile and prescribe what is needed. Most parents would agree that they have their own bag of tricks that children grow to respect and appreciate. I adapt this model to a professional metaphor such as a doctor's bag. It works, and it sounds more acceptable than a psychiatrist's couch. My doctor's bag includes hope, support, smiles, grins, and sometimes a simple perspective to allow others to look at life a little differently.

Another point to remember is the importance of knowing how much is too much when prescribing humor. Start where someone is (assessment), and then facilitate his or her humor. Too much humor makes you appear like a clown trying to attract attention. It's truly a better, intrinsic feeling when you've made a difference, and the credit goes to the situation, not to the clown.

Humor therapy is two-directional and interactive. It requires a conversation between two people so humor can surface on its own. Humor is massaged and nurtured to allow it to find its place in our conversations, and training and practice are required to do this. Do not think that a single joke will make someone feel better. Instead, talk to a person about his or her most embarrassing moments, funniest vacation, or funniest birthday party. This promotes two-directional humor at its best, and it leaves a residue that is remembered longer. Other ways to promote two-directional humor include board games that offer opportunities to laugh during play, talking about silly things you have seen your pet do, and finding common ground in all things around you.

Most humor experienced today is one-directional. A comic gets on a stage and throws humor at us. It is then up to us to laugh in response. If the comic stops telling jokes, we stop laughing. He is in control of our humor. This isn't a bad thing, but it trains us to look at humor through his eyes, not ours. TV sitcoms, comic strips, movies, and jokesters are usually one-directional. They deliver; we receive.

Conversation is the best delivery vehicle for humor therapy with positive human interaction being the core of its success. Humor therapy is also a prescribed moment or thought with the pure intent of healing and inspiring others. It's not about the joke at hand. It's about the connection and communication that is shared through humor.

The following great example is from Carol Brooks, a retired teacher and incredible volunteer at one of the Serious Fun Children's Network therapeutic camps founded by Paul Newman:

> At camp one weekend, I had a new camper who said he couldn't do anything well!
>
> I tried to get him interested in some new things and he mentioned he liked "putt-putt" but couldn't really do it because of his wheelchair. At camp that doesn't matter. Off to the mini golf course we went. When he asked me if I knew how to play I told him I didn't. He said he would be my teacher and had a big smile on his face. At the first hole I, of course, approached the ball doing everything wrong I could think of. He gave me a strange look and allowed me to continue. Fifteen strokes and he said, "I have a lot of work to do!" The whole family and I laughed so hard. Hole number two I was given all of the right instructions, every little detail was covered. I hit the ball and it went straight in the hole. He looked at me with his big blue eyes and shaggy blonde hair

and said, "Wow, Carol, I am a fantastic teacher aren't I? I didn't know I could teach so well." After many smiles, side hugs and big high fives, we finished the round. Of course he won! After putting up the clubs he looked at me and said, "You know what? If I can teach you to play golf, I can do anything!" That he did. He tried everything new and had a wonderful weekend full of many laughs and excitement.

The real trick is to intentionally and purposefully know where you are taking a person in need before you speak. It must be slightly positive and uplifting, so humor can organically grow on its own. Believe in your tools and you will be more effective.

For example, I might take a friend out to lunch who has just gone through something that has caused him grief, concern, and worry. My job is to spend time with that person and provide something that gives relief and maybe a little comfort. It may even be my responsibility to help him escape from the moment and take a fresh look at life. No easy task, I know, but who but a friend can do it better? We talk over lunch, and I see that if I let my friend take the lead on the conversation, it goes downward and slightly negative. He is still dealing with the issues at hand. I provide active listening skills and nod at the right moments. I say "I see" and "That's right," and sometimes I add "I hear you." But when it is my turn to pivot the conversation to a new direction, I must be ready to pull him into it and not appear to be insensitive to where his mind has drifted. I believe that this is best done with compassion and careful timing.

Being sincere and taking advantage of the precise pause, you can reach into your doctor's bag and pull out something that reminds him of why you are such a great friend. It may be something as simple as a comment such as: "Wow, that reminds me of the time you and I got cake on our Sunday school clothes and ..." Or it could be an "Oh, I almost forgot to tell you what happened to me yesterday" story. Even a cute pet story can redirect someone in a pinch.

Knowing the direction of the conversation is like racing turtles in a one-turtle race down a track. You keep slightly pointing them in the right direction while following them down the track. Sometimes you do not even touch the turtle; other times you turn it forty-five degrees. Success is not in having your turtle beat other turtles but in crossing the finish line with a few grins, snickers, and smiles. The turtle may know you turned it a few times but does not mind because the trip was filled with your support. Too much guiding can cause the turtle to stop, and no turtle likes that. It withdraws into its shell, and no one gets to the finish line. Remember, *do no harm.*

Do you recall the game of pitching pennies? Each person gets a turn and the goal is to toss your penny as close as possible to the wall. If your penny hits the wall or bounces into it, your pitch does not count and the other guy wins. The way to win is to toss it just the right amount, just short of touching the wall.

The best penny pitchers are the ones who develop the skills to be accurately precise without ever going too far. All under-pitched pennies are still in the game and counted.

The same is true with people's feelings. Too much control and too much leading can cause your input to be discounted. Less control can keep you in the game of lifting spirits and morale.

When I think of ways to help with humor, I always come back to the soda machine story.

Imagine you see a youth in front of a soda machine. He is very frustrated by the fact that he just put in the correct amount of change and is getting nothing from the machine. You can tell by his body language and the steam coming out of his ears that he is not happy.

At this very moment, before he starts kicking the machine, you have a great opportunity to help the situation and interact with positive support. Approaching the machine, you see that the lights are not on.

He might not have noticed this due to the fact that it is midday and the lights are not that noticeable. You suspect that the machine is not plugged in, is out of order, or the electricity is out.

You could use sarcasm and simply point out what he has missed by saying something like "Do you often try to get something out of a vending machine that's not on?" Nothing is gained with this method except making yourself feel better by thinking you are smarter than others, and pointing it out solidifies a superior attitude. Or you could use this opportunity to share an important altruistic moment. Here's how. Instead of pointing out the obvious by humiliating the youth, ask if you may help. At this precise moment, suggest he look at the total machine to see if something else is going on with the machine. Send him to the side where the electrical cord plugs into the outlet allowing him to discover the power issue. You might ask, "Can you tell if there are any lights on?" During the conversation and up to the point of discovery is the time frame to build the relationship. Think of it as a sort of cordial small talk with patience on your side. No doubt he will discover the problem as you support his need to get to the final result, a can of soda. The precise second that he reaches the "Aha!" moment, you can mirror his humor to his comfort level. He will then add his own splash of humor and bring closure to the problem. All along, the goal of this interaction was to help with frustrations by bringing a bucket of warmhearted feelings for him to use on himself.

It doesn't matter if the machine is unplugged or out of order. Reach into your pocket for a few coins and help him with his loss. The kind act, the warm light humor, and the interaction are worth a million bucks.

Remember, feelings can be stepped on in the course of getting a laugh. By sprinkling a little humor, helping others discover solutions, and being present in the moment of any and all issues, you are creating a memory for others to look back on years from now. Plus, the memory just might prompt a smile as they retell the story.

In problem situations, humor allows one to seek ways to help without taking over or adding more discomfort to others.

As a camp director many years ago, I added a small line drawing of a ladder on all of the counselor staff shirts. It was placed right below the camp logo on the front of each shirt. The counselors were cool enough to make up their explanations when campers asked what it meant. Some stated that it represented reaching for heights unknown or something about getting to the top of things. Some even described the ladder imprint as a tool for getting a higher perspective on things. The true meaning, which was described during their staff training prior to the camp, was that it represented a tool to help others.

Picture a child getting into trouble for any given reason. Figuratively, he digs himself into a hole. Most would say the first thing to do is tell him to stop digging. That's good advice, but it does not offer the next step of how to get out of the hole. If we imagine carrying around a pretend ladder in our pockets, we could pull it out when we see others in need. With ladder in hand, we peer down into the deep hole, and instead of saying, "What were you thinking? You are in a hole now!" you could show support from above. Then you could lower your ladder into the hole, climb down, and talk to the child. During this effort, you would most likely calm and soothe the child's worries. Now, the important part is that you don't pick him up and climb back out with him on your shoulder like a sack of potatoes. Instead, you help him climb out on his own, one ladder rung at a time. Along the climb, you provide support and praise so he can begin to master his own problems. If done correctly, a handful of opportunities will present themselves for humor to surface.

A lot of people use humor to laugh off mistakes and serious issues they face. It appears as nervous laughter or inappropriate giggling. These are moments that I look for so I can slightly reinforce their humor or even guide them to a healthy means of expressing themselves. Keep in mind that when someone is struggling or encountering a problem that is taking all their focus, your strategic and indirect support of humor is by far more effective than simply pointing out the funny side of their problem. In fact, humor can be the bright side of misery that occurs if self-discovered. You also have to ask yourself if the point is to be the first to notice something or the first to help with it. It's just that simple.

Want a real life example? Okay, here's something you can do. Keep jumper cables in your car for when you see another motorist in need, such as someone in a big box store parking lot whose car lights were left on too long and the battery has drained. Simply retrieve the cables and assist. Notice how your interactions come into play as much as having the jumper cables do. The opportunity here is to help that person find humor in the situation and lift his spirits through positive conversation. The cables also allow for a quick pun when needed: "You are not starting something with others, are you?"

Imaginary ladders or real jumper cables—the point is that if you have them, you'll be more likely to seek others in need and use them.

Think about it this way: if someone you care about was in pain from a life crisis or feeling profoundly low from daily issues and you truly wanted to help, what would you do? You might consider spending some time with him or taking him out for an evening getaway. Or you might even consider inviting him along with a few of his friends over for dinner, friends who would add a little positive cheer to the gathering. Imagine that your plans are in motion, and there you are— sitting there with nothing to say. Well, don't just let the conversation wither without trying this: just be there for him.

It happens to be quite easy if you have invested time prior to that person's need. The relationship is already rich with memories of better days, funny experiences, and things you encountered together. Be there when needed and allow the humor to organically grow. While feeling down, he will smile at himself at some point and realize that it could be worse. Helping him feel comfortable during the process is sometimes all you can do. Otherwise, you might appear to be trying too hard. And remember—it is acceptable to just share space with him with no conversation. Your presence alone is comforting to a true friend.

Talk about neutral things, gravitate toward the positive, and slightly lean to the humorous perspective of the situation. When the conversation goes sour, be patient and do not add to the negative validation of his words. Just pause and start again with positive support through kind words. Past generations would simply say, "There, there." Today's culture is a bit more complex, but the concept is the same by simply saying, "I'm here for you."

Here is yet another way to look at it. A feather will always fall downward as gravity pulls on it, but you can keep it afloat if you gently blow on its underside. Too much winded effort can cause you to pass out, and not enough wind will allow the feather to hit the ground. Just the right amount of wind (love and support) will keep a friend in midair and allow her to discover what she needs. When the moment arrives and she says something (anything) that prompts a smile or chuckle, validate the moment and mirror the mood. Don't go overboard and snap back with an over-the-top joke or change the subject, but just smile for her and match her effort. This whole attempt takes time, and it's about waiting for her to advance toward humor at her pace. You are the facilitator of positive slow-growth humor. Nobody likes a clown to walk up and start making funny expressions while juggling when he or she is not ready for it. It can be overwhelming. The dialogue between two friends can ease even the worst of situations given time together. You've heard the saying that a problem shared is half as bad, while a joy shared is twice as good. It's the same principle here.

If the setting has humor potential, then you have the opportunity to incorporate this into the conversation. Settings like the park, a zoo, a front porch, or a mall food court work well. An office cubicle, an empty hallway, or confined quarters do not assist in creating smiles. If you can't change the environment for whatever reason, then change the immediate surroundings with immediate stimuli: look through a yearbook and comment on the fashions, surf through animal pictures on the Internet and seek critters that look like family members, flip through family albums and add captions and comments to them, or look at clouds and spot animal shapes or cartoons.

Opportunities to have dialogue in a lighthearted atmosphere give you more control to be the natural wind beneath a friend's feather and allow you to pause and support as needed. Parents know this best when they nurture their children by adding sugar and spice to their children's humor growth when needed. But they also allow snakes, snails, and puppy-dog tails to sneak in an unexpected laugh. Think ahead, plan the environment, and just be there for your friend.

When things do go silent and you find yourself struggling to come up with things to talk about, prep yourself with a humor conversation tool. Simply visualize and memorize the following story. Included is a reference key to remind you of the conversation topics. It can be useful during one-on-one interactions or small group discussions.

This is a great mental model to use in the future to start conversations with anyone, participate in small talk, and cultivate opportunities for smiles and laughter.

Story

You are walking down a road when you see a gingerbread house. A mailbox shaped like a large gumdrop has some writings on it. You walk to the front door and notice several types of comfortable chairs on the front porch. Before you sit on one, the door opens and you look inside. In front of you is a mantel with family photos of events, festivals, and birthday parties. On a side table, there are two concert tickets and a vacation brochure. There is a clown's nose on the floor. You trip over it and laugh out loud.

Key

Gingerbread house: What kind of place do you live in? Anything novel or unique about it?

Gumdrop mailbox: What kind of sweets do you crave? Funny neighbors?
Comfortable chairs: Favorite place to sit for the view? Beach chairs, swing, or patio furniture?
Family photos: Memorable family gatherings or reunions? Pets?
Festivals and birthday parties: Fun outings or festive gatherings?
Concert tickets: Music or plays?
Vacation brochure: Favorite vacation or getaway?
Clown's nose: What makes you laugh? Sitcoms? Comic strips? Kittens?
You trip: Embarrassing moments? Mishaps you'll never forget?
Laugh out loud: When was the last time you did this?

When there is a long pause or silent moment that lingers too long during a conversation, mentally put yourself into the story and ask questions about each key visual you memorized. Just pick and choose any key. Use what is relevant for the situation. For instance, talking to someone about where he or she is from is positive and polite but not needed if you already know this information. Skip to asking about leisure opportunities, festivals, and family events.

If you get lost and hung up with where the conversation should go next, just choose another key and explore more lighthearted stuff. Conversations like this always bring a smile or two.

So how do we spread humor in a more positive way? Simply train yourself to view humor as something special, and share it with as many people as possible. It's like a rainbow. Once a rainbow is spotted in the sky, it is true human nature to look around and see who has not spotted it. We want to share the moment with others quickly before it disappears. Once shared, we always smile at each other, nod with a compassionate spark in our eyes, and feel better about ourselves. I believe that this works because humans have a basic need to share in a positive way. Similar to a rainbow, humor is pleasing to share.

If you train yourself to notice the beauty of things, you slowly become more positive in all your interactions with others. Humor leaves a residue that is hard to explain. Notice others' reactions next time you share a great family story about something that made you laugh. Oral histories in our family trees are still the most powerful ways to demonstrate and perpetuate one's sense of humor.

Any time I notice someone's mishap, I wait just a few seconds before interjecting a comment. Timing is paramount in helping others feel better. If you say something too soon, you come across as a jokester looking for attention at the expense of other's misfortunes. If you wait too long, on the other hand, you miss the opportunity to maximize a healing effort.

Many times when I witness a waitress drop something in front of me, I simply smile, wait a few seconds to insure my comment will not add to the misery or embarrassment, and supportively say something like, "You okay?" She usually follows with a small grin and apology. If the mood is neutral or anywhere positive in nature, I then state, "Cool, thanks for the entertainment!" I know this seems very small as a humor opportunity, but it is not measured in your perspective of the problem as much as it is measured in the human connection and allowing humor to surface on its own. Much to my surprise, situations like this usually prompt wait staff to come back later to continue a conversation that is warm, friendly, and just ever so slightly funny. Ask yourself a basic question during these situations—"Who is the victim and how can I help?" If I start there, a supportive atmosphere is created and humor surfaces to the top like cream. I have taught myself to never say something like "Good move, Grace" when I observe mishaps. This comment always promotes a laugh from others, as it has been around for decades, but it just sends a negative comment to the victim and labels him or her as inferior. It's too easy to look at this comment as just a funny insult, but it could also be described as an intentional blow to someone's confidence or self-esteem. The fork in the road is best decided after waiting a few seconds, assessing the situation, and moving forward with the best option for all involved. My intent is to sprinkle these moments with light humor or, even better, to create opportunities for others to add humor themselves.

Remember—empathy is about sharing a feeling with someone, as opposed to sympathy and feeling pity for that person. Patient observation and attentiveness to situations sets the stage for positive outcomes. Follow this correctly, and you will find yourself being more intuitive about the whole conversation.

If there is one dedicated agenda I follow daily, it's bringing a smile to my wife (extra bonus if it's a laugh). This is done through making small silly statements; pointing out life's silly treasures; admiring the ridiculous; redirecting stress; adding sound effects to normal sights; ribbing our relationship; asking fun questions; sharing humor moments from our day; exchanging our wedding bands unexpectedly while she leaves it on the dresser; asking questions that promote funny answers; pretending we just met; looking for moments that promote winking at each other; grabbing her hand on the way into a store and saying, "Come with me little one"; nudging her shoulder after saying something cute; smiling at her with puppy-dog eyes after messing up something; being supportive when she messes up something while I jump in quickly and pretend that it was all my mistake; leaving a Post-it note on her mirror in the bathroom that says "You are cute, but please comb your hair"; and, most of all, saying "I love you" in as many creative, fun ways I can come up with.

We laugh at the absurdities of life, people-watch together, take cooking classes together, enjoy wine festivals, play little harmless jokes on each other, and enjoy each moment as a unique opportunity to share a laugh.

So what does all of this have to do with humor therapy? Everything. Humor is just another heart-to-heart connection that humans have. If a tool is offered to enhance that connection, I say use it. Start smiling for others, and show people that you are interested in what they have to say. This sets the platform for humor to grow organically in a nonjudgmental atmosphere.

Try This:

Remember a time when you had a cast on one of your limbs or maybe a Band-Aid on a visible spot? It seems like you instantly notice everyone else in the world with a cast or Band-Aid. Or have you ever bought a new car and all of a sudden you notice all the cars of the same make and model? It is amazing how we as humans often seek out or notice things that are similar to us or in the same situation. There is scientific research of this, but that is for another book. Anyway, it's there. Take advantage of this human behavior to notice the sunny side of life. On any given day, look for funny sights, humorous pictures, and things that are out of place. Each time you see something; force yourself to chuckle or smile inside. And, whenever possible, point it out and share with others. Your day will be filled with zest—guaranteed. As I suggested before, share your rainbows whenever possible.

A word of caution here. Please do not train yourself to laugh at others in this activity. This includes the way people walk, their appearance, or any misfortunes they encounter. Keep your humor visuals 100 percent positive. This will prevent you from falling into the "superior over others" mentality, which nobody likes. Good luck out there.

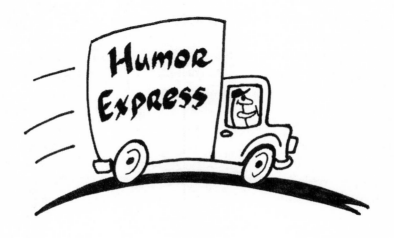

Laughing like this is just as nice as anything we could be doing anywhere else right now.

CHAPTER 4

BEING CHILDISH VS. CHILDLIKE

While in graduate school at Clemson University, I had the pleasure of taking a class presented by Ann James, PhD, on humor therapy. This included many research-backed models, humor concepts, clown therapy, and hospital room visits. We learned the basics of how humor heals as well as how it hurts if used in the wrong way. I had been to a variety of hospital wards singing Christmas songs to patients prior to taking her class, but one major lesson I learned from her was how to seek a connection prior to entering a hospital room. It reminded me of the example of pitching pennies, as I described in the last chapter. Go slow, and never do harm when humor is involved.

First of all, it does not matter if you are wearing a clown outfit or street clothes. It also does not matter if you already know the person or it's the first time you are meeting him or her. Stop and pause in the doorway of a patient's room. Look into the patient's eyes. If his eyes are closed or not looking your way, say in a calm, low tone, "Hello." This will initiate eye contact. Once you have that, give a warm heartfelt smile and check for what I call an *eye spark*. Follow your instinct and determine if that spark is due to his welcoming you in, or if it is due to pain and suffering. In your best guess, choose one of the following two options.

1) His eye spark is due to pain and misery, and/or he appears sad or stressed.

Proceed slowly with sincere compassion and try to verbally connect. Follow his lead and do not throw humor at him such as juggling, laughing, or joke telling.

Pretend to leave your imaginary doctor's bag on the floor, and look for reasons later to use it. At this moment, a simple "I'm here to brighten your day. How can I help?" is enough. Your work may be cut out for you due to the patient being in a miserable state, but you will still make a difference. Remember, the imaginary doctor's bag is always within reach. Use it when the timing is right.

2) His eye spark has a sparkle of hope and gleams of wanting to be uplifted.

Proceed slowly with making merry and demonstrating as much positive zest as you can. The patient has been waiting for something like this all day. His eye spark will instantly be followed by a smile, and this is your opportunity to interact with healing humor. Grab that imaginary doctor's bag and go at it.

The important point here is to consider the patient's goals and needs. It should be his call if the hospital room is spontaneously filled with entertainment or not. And as always, if in doubt, proceed slowly until you know more. Remember *assessment* from chapter 2?

During my childhood years, a friend and I would occasionally visit his grandfather and sit on the front porch looking out at the small neighborhood. We would just sit there and talk about life and the absurdities of living in a small town. His grandfather would usually plan a simple joke or slide a humor item into the conversation in some strange yet delightful way. I recall one day walking up to the porch and noticing that he was smoking an extremely long tobacco pipe. The stem must have been at least a foot long. He was just lighting it as we approached, probably his plan. We kept staring at his long pipe as the conversation circled around topics involving the weather, dinner, and his work projects. He was being circumloquacious (yes, this is a real word) as he avoided commenting and talking in circles about his new pipe. Finally, after several snickers and elbowing each other, we asked, "So what's with the long-stem pipe?" This was the moment he was priming us for as he boldly stated, "Doctor's orders. He told me to stay as far away from tobacco as I could." We hooted out loud and treasured this humor moment for years.

His sense of humor was subtle, low key, and polite. He would plan ahead and with precision inject just what was needed to highlight his humor prescription for us.

I often used this soft-prop type of humor in my hospital room visits by simply carrying in a gag prop and not saying what it was until they asked me about it. Items included a square dry sponge with *add water* written on its side. At some point I would pull it out and ask, "Wanna see something swell?" Or a large piece of felt that I would pull out of a pocket and state, "This is how I felt yesterday." Or showing two bananas that were *a pair of slippers*. Or presenting a cheap jump rope and saying, "This is for ... oh skip it." Or my favorite one was the curly piece of wire between a phone base and the hand held portion of a phone, just the twelve inches of curly wire. "What is this? Oh just my new phone-less cord." Whatever you use, please remember to keep it positive.

Nowadays when I provide training sessions for camp counselors, pediatric nurses, or role model workshops, I always reinforce that positive humor heals and negative humor hurts. If you watch most of today's TV sitcoms you will notice that laugh tracks assist in making the unfunny funny. Their humor includes about 80 percent negative put downs, sarcasm, and insults. We hear negative comedy with a roar of laughter and think it is okay to laugh at inappropriate situations and the misfortune of others. I believe that a whole generation has developed a negative sense of humor because of this.

Back in the day, Don Rickles was the king of insults. It was funny because his humor was different from the norm and somewhat shocking. Not always considered politically correct, his humor was justified by the fact that he left no ethnic group out. Everyone was the butt of his jokes. Today, negative humor is the norm, and one can see its influence in our youth's interactions. They don't share jokes; they throw jokes and punch lines at one another and hope it sticks. Ever heard someone say *bazinga* or *burn*?

Once upon a time I loved this one. I would simply ask a young camper, "Want to hear a dirty joke?" The camper's eager response would always be similar to "Sure!" I then proudly answered, "A clean horse fell into a mud hole." Ninety percent of the time I used this joke, the camper would return later that day with a *real* dirty joke. I finally retired this one, knowing that if you even suggest the gutter, you open the door for more gutter. Hence, as an adult role model, I share only corny clean humor to all I encounter. I may get groans and sound effects, but they leave smiling and sometimes say, "Ha, good one."

Often I ask participants, "Does anyone have a clean positive joke they can share?"

The responses sometimes shock me. One participant replied, "Why did the monkey fall from the tree?" The punch line was "Because he was dead." I politely tried to explain why that joke was funny in the right group setting of adults but was probably not the best joke for the young campers of oncology week at that particular therapeutic facility.

I also heard, "Did you hear about the lawyer, the pastor, and the____?" I usually have to cut them off before they can finish because this standard joke type usually offends someone.

I then challenge the group to share only positive, corny yet clean jokes with the crowd. This is not easy for most people because they don't know any. I suggest they seek out sources, like paperback books of clean jokes for kids, *Readers Digest* humor, and websites that have clean positive humor. A favorite of mine is: "There are three types of people in this world, those that can count and those that can't."

Test time: Is this joke okay?

A skeleton walks into a bar and asks, "Can I have a shot of whiskey and a mop?"

Or this one: "Did you hear about the dyslexic atheist that did not believe in a dog?"

And last but not least, this one: "How many bullies does it take to screw in a light bulb?" Answer: "Three. You got a problem with that?"

When you analyze these jokes, it's clear that in some form or another, they either offend someone or bring up an adult content conversation. It is best not to tell bar jokes to youth. Dyslexia is a learning disability and not cool to joke about. Bullying is a hot topic in schools and camps across our country and also not a joking matter.

Now don't get me wrong here. I find myself at times laughing at inappropriate humor. The difference is that as a humor therapist, I have trained myself to be a role model who knows that every word that comes out of my mouth can and will be heard—and will often be repeated. Hence the reason I usually go with puns and silly conversations. They fit into an already ongoing conversation directed toward a positive outcome.

With a clean sense of humor that is childlike and not childish, I'm reminded of the human response every time I hear a particular joke. It goes something like this:

Q: What happened when the owl lost his voice?
A: He didn't give a hoot!

The normal response is one of the following (some with sound effects and some with hand motions):

Ahhhh.
Ooooo.
Wacka wacka wacka.

Ba da dum.
Waaaa Waaaa.
*Groooaaa*n.
Stares with an unspoken *I'm not taking the bait.*
Really?

They may show no reaction, stare, bite their lip, or maybe roll their eyes a little just to demonstrate their superiority to your attempt at humor. But remember this; being childlike is okay while being childish is not always okay.

But sometimes they give a courtesy laugh, which is okay in my book.

All of these responses dismiss the child in us and allow the adult in us to maintain posture, retain maturity, and not appear childish— important qualities if you are very serious-minded. I tend to think that these general responses prompt those around us to view humor as secondary or just downright silly. When adults laugh out loud, grin, or even giggle a bit after a pun or simple joke, they reinforce to the joke teller that the effort was good, appreciated, and even encouraged. Negative responses like the ones listed above are echoed by other adults within listening range. It seems to spread quickly through the mind-set of those who don't have time for such silliness. How sad that these same people are missing out on one of the best human experiences of all, humor at the basic level.

So the next time a child tells you a joke, laugh; even if you know the punch line, laugh out loud. Remember, it's not about you. It's about that child trying out humor techniques and practicing humor styles. It's also about reaching out to share something funny. Your only job is to receive and show appreciation through laughter. You will reinforce the child's humor development that will carry him or her through life.

Oh yes, allow me to share an inside scoop here: this works with adults too.

What about sarcasm?

Is sarcasm negative or mean-spirited? Or is there more to it? Melanie Wilbur, a close friend, and I would debate this often. I would state that sarcasm is a way to say, "You just did something stupid and I'm going to make fun of you with my next comment." Melanie would state that sarcasm is best used for "breaking the ice, easing the tension, lightening the mood, and even addressing the elephant in the room to get people to feel more relaxed about an obvious and possibly uncomfortable situation. These are all things that can be done without mean sarcasm. Even if it's just a smile or a laugh to break the ice, I feel like that's not a bad thing."

I have come to the conclusion that her arguments have validity, and now I view sarcasm as a useful tool in humor therapy if used correctly. In its simplest form, sarcasm can be demonstrated with the question, "Hot enough for you?" while smiling on a hot day.

Melanie further states:

> Quite simply, my point about sarcasm is that it's like any other type of humor. It can hurt someone and be used to make fun of someone, or it can lighten the mood and be an icebreaker if used in a correct way. For example, stating the obvious in a dry way can be considered sarcasm (it usually is), but in a tense situation or a nervous situation, it could be just the thing that lightens the mood and gets people smiling and/or talking. They may be "zingers," "one-liners," or "Ooh, BURN," but they can also be witty, clever, and funny without being at someone's expense as well. I like to think of sarcasm as dry humor with a pinch of extra wit for good measure. If the sarcasm is used to make light of a situation, rather than make fun of a person, it can really put people at ease. Is it mean? Yes, if used that way. It's a lot more than saying something mean and then saying "just kidding," which is how a lot of people interpret sarcasm. In fact, that's not sarcasm or humor at all. That's just saying something mean, realizing it went too far or sounded too mean, and then trying to play it off before you look like a total jerk. It's one of those forms of

humor (because I believe it is) that can also help a person accept something, whether they say it about themselves or to someone else. Sarcasm is a great way to address "the elephant in the room" in a relaxed way that can put people at ease.

It takes the awkward out of a situation in a very direct, yet (done correctly) funny way. It doesn't get a "fair shake" because people typically use, and are accustomed to, the mean "zingers." It's more than that. It's hard to even find good examples of sarcasm on the Internet, because most people go to the mean, one-liners. I think that this is hurt by the fact that Oxford Dictionary has quite a unique origin for the word: "sarcasm" derives from ancient Greek for "to tear flesh, gnash the teeth, speak bitterly." Its first definition is "a sharp, bitter, or cutting expression or remark; a bitter gibe or taunt."

(Yikes!) This is the general perception of sarcasm, however.

The comic strip character Garfield is very sarcastic, yet not (always) mean. Another example: You and your classmates show up for class. The door is locked, the lights are off, and after you finally get inside (after having called security and waiting for them to unlock the door), you feel that the temperature is very uncomfortably hot. You say, "Ah, it was so nice of them to prepare the room for our class today, wasn't it? I mean, it isn't like they knew this class was scheduled all semester or anything." It's not mean, and you'll get typically, one of two reactions: Either a laugh or an "I know, right?!" which sparks a conversation. Just like the kid who trips someone for laughs, sarcasm also has a mean side (as all humor does). But it does have a different, albeit, less utilized side as well.

Sarcasm is an art form. In the right situation or with the right people it is fun (as with all humor, you should know your audience). No one feels insulted because you are all able to laugh at yourself and are comfortable laughing with each other. It's also a way to combat ignorance, negativity, or rudeness. Sometimes it DOES stop people and put them in their place, but when used right, it's because they need it. It IS a specialized science! Of course, like any humor, it can be used to hurt, but when perfected, it can ease tension, break ice, and create laughter. It's about timing, delivery, and appropriateness.

Sarcasm is stating the obvious in a way that people can find humor in it and allows one to laugh at themselves or with each other. It is simply one's unwillingness to find humor in things that makes true sarcasm unfunny.

As you can see, Melanie has great perspective on sarcasm, and she uses it in a positive, helpful manner. Her views have changed my perspective, and I now feel that it can comfortably fit into the humor therapy model described in this book.

What do you think? In your own experience, has sarcasm been hurtful or has it been an icebreaker? Have you experienced it both ways? Knowing what makes those around you laugh can be helpful when it comes to deciding if sarcasm will be helpful or hurtful. In today's world of quick laughs and negative humor, one should be careful. If nothing else, those around you will help keep you in check if you cross the line and offend someone.

What about gallows or dark humor?

This is a type of humor used in select settings and environments. It is a cognitive and behavioral coping strategy that sometimes is a reaction to stressful events and situations. Imagine your local emergency room staff, day after day, seeing gruesome sights, blood, wounds, and horrors of the human condition. Their sense of humor is often quite gloomy and morbid. Most professional medical employees share this type of humor with each other at some time or another as they use it to de-stress and make sense of their daily duties. You can also imagine other professions such as undertakers, surgeons, and port-a-potty transporters who share such dark humor.

Working in a therapeutic camp, many counselors would throw *poopie parties.* Covering themselves from head to toe with latex gloves, gowns, and footsies, they assisted many campers with their bowel movements and bathroom routines at night. To help ease and comfort the campers, a party would be thrown and music played while laughter was the common language. Only then would the following jokes be shared.

Q. What is the difference between toilet paper and toast?
A. Toast is brown on both sides.

Q. Did you hear about the elephant with diarrhea?
A. It's all over town.

Q. Do you know how to cook toilet paper?
A. Throw it in a pot and brown one side.

Keep in mind that these counselors would never share any of these jokes with campers outside this specific situation. It was prescribed when needed and nothing more. But in the hearts of campers with serious intestinal illnesses, this humor was often just what the doctor ordered.

I bring up this type of humor to remind you that—just like sarcasm—gallows humor is a serious humor therapy tool. It is best used only if you are in certain groups where it can be prescribed. Otherwise, use it only when you are 100 percent sure that you will be doing no harm.

Try This:

An activity that my lovely wife and I came up with can be enjoyed in any environment. It's called *Look at that, what do you see?* While walking anywhere—short hikes into nature is our favorite—take turns and leisurely take the time to notice something novel or unique within your sight line. Point to it and say, "Look at that, what do you see?" The other person then responds, keeping it lighthearted, funny, creative, or zany. Simply make up something out of the blue. An example might be viewing a flat rock with moss growing on one side of it and a small stick leaning over its corner. After the obvious question is asked, a sample response could be something like, "I see a bearded face with a toothpick in his mouth and he's singing 'Row, Row, Row your boat.'"

Viewing a knot on a tree trunk could be a door keyhole viewer for gnomes hiding inside. A piece of dirt clod could be a miniature anchor for a beetle's sailboat. The sillier the better, even if it's a stretch.

Take turns with a slow pace, allowing the sights to come easily and not be forced. And most of all, remember that the goal is to keep the activity lighthearted and slightly humorous. You will be surprised to find that the game gets funnier as you go. It also teaches one to look at the funny side of life where others miss out.

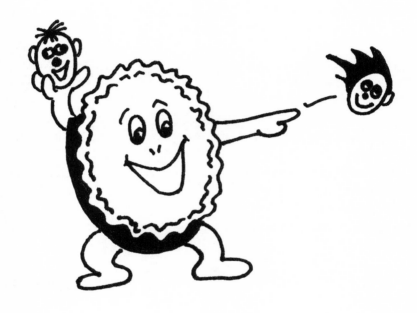

If it is not your nature to be funny, then just be a
little funny-natured when others need it.

Chapter 5

QUESTIONS, ANSWERS, AND QUOTES

The following section contains the thoughts, comments, and quotes of others who understand the concepts of humor therapy.

1) In your own words, what is humor therapy?

Humor therapy is not about baking cookies and giving them to someone. It's about sharing the cookies and laughing together.
—Debbie Mann, artist and illustrator

Humor therapy is similar to smiling. Smiling for yourself is easy and sometimes automatic. Smiling for others requires giving of yourself with purposeful intent.
—David Smith, performing arts director, Robert M. Cooper Leadership Center

Humor therapy is the art of healing through laughter, jokes and joy.
—Crystal Emerick, marketing and PR consultant

To me humor therapy means providing an outlet for others to laugh and smile. Whether that is making a fool of yourself or setting someone else up with a joke that will bring smiles to them and others.
—Rocco Richard, recreation program supervisor, Chatham County Parks and Recreation

Helping someone to have a laugh to overcome an issue, getting their mind off the issue they are dealing with at that point and time. Help them feel good.
—Thomas L. Olsen

Humor therapy is a two-way street. Drive slow at first and avoid head on collisions. Along your travels, you just might help others feel better about *their* driving skills.
—Walt Willis

Using laughter to help heal whatever is ailing someone!
—Claire Rutan

Funny things never get the respect they deserve. Humor, if provided in the proper form, makes all of us feel better inside and out. It's been my experience that funny people are much better at providing humor therapy for others than prescribing it for themselves. In the end I believe that humor therapy is about social awareness. When you are aware of how you can positively (or negatively) affect the world around you, you have an easier time finding the simple things in life that are funny or humorous. The therapeutic part is simply the act of sharing it with others.
—Pronto Parenteau

Humor therapy is pulling out of your pocket that one happy moment that you know will bring a smile to someone's face.
—Cindy Handley

Being able to make people feel good about themselves and not think about their problems.
—Pat Stubbs, national secretary for the Volunteer Outreach Network; president of the West Virginia Community Educational Outreach Service

Dealing with stressful situations through laughter.
—Patti Brown

Humor therapy is a deliberate attempt to bring playfulness and the ability to laugh into an environment.
—Stavros Michailidis

2) Share an example of when you have prescribed humor to someone in need of a smile or laugh.

After the funeral of a close friend, a few of us gathered off to the side and just stood there silently looking at each other, absorbed in our own thoughts. I kept thinking of the many funny moments of our dear friend's life. There just wasn't the right time to bring them up. I finally said, "You guys feel like I do? I don't know whether to laugh or cry. I miss him so much. His smile would always make my day. How about you guys?" What followed was an hour of amazing funny memories involving our dear lost friend. We truly celebrated his life and how he rubbed off on all of us.
—David Smith, performing arts director, Robert M. Cooper Leadership Center

I am a high school sports official. Sometimes the coaches don't agree with your calls. If a coach is walking out to question or complain to you, he is figuring out what he is going to say as he is walking. I try to break his train of thought by asking him an unexpected question just before he gets to me. He usually has to redirect his entire train of thought and the conversation doesn't last very long.
—Todd Moore and Janet Moore

The very first summer at camp my unit had the youngest kids. It was our turn to go to the fab shop (camp's version of a beauty salon) and the boys were a little disappointed. Makeup is for girls!!!! Once we got in there and they saw the girls painting my nails and putting makeup on the other male counselors, they went nuts. For the rest of the week all they wanted to do was go to the fab shop and make us look silly. It made their week and it made my summer.
—Rocco Richard, recreation program supervisor, Chatham County Parks and Recreation

A dear friend of mine had just lost her husband to cancer and was having a hard time with the loss. I had just returned from camp where I attended Sunday service lead by David Mann. He had explained how

getting people to "rub elbows" was good humor medicine. I used this technique and with a smile on her face she asked, "What are you doing?" I rubbed our elbows again and she continued to smile. I kept doing it and she asked, "Why are you doing this?" I said, "You're smiling aren't you?" She said, "Yes," and then "Thank you." She had a smile on her face for the rest of the day. This occurred at work and everyone was wondering why she was smiling. When asked she said to them, "Because."
—Thomas L. Olsen

As a camp director I prescribe humor on a daily basis as a way of making others more comfortable around me. When a child finds themselves in a crisis situation and they are not in complete control of their behavior, I use humor as a sort of litmus test to see when the child is ready to rejoin the group. Humor breaks the ice and makes an uncomfortable situation, like behavior modification, more enjoyable and memorable. The end goal is to use humor as the lasting memory or final thought when you are trying to get an important point across to an individual. I've also had to use humor therapy a number of times when delivering bad news to staff or volunteer, specifically a death in the family. Initially the news is devastating and causes the person grief and even pain, but I like to sit and process with the person until we can enter a place where we remember their loved one fondly. Eventually you'll find that the conversation leads you to a place where you can remember something funny that they did. The point is that we remember the loved one's humorous side and when they were happy. That humor helps us to heal.
—Pronto Parenteau

My husband and I used to go to an occasional concert with our pastor Bob Bender and his wife Jane. I would always say that Bob was such a Sandi Patty groupie! They would drive long distances just to see Sandi Patty in concert over and over again. He passed away a few years ago. So now whenever I see that Jane is down, I go up to her and start talking about how much of a "groupie" Bob was and all the fun we had going to some of the concerts. It always puts a smile on her face.
—Cindy Handley

I am very involved in the Red Hat society. We were having some problems and having a hard time with attendance and some sick members. At this year's Christmas party, we needed to get everyone into the swing of things and have fun, so this year we decided to do something different and dress up as our favorite Christmas songs. There was "Silent Night" and "Rudolph" and so on. But I decided to go completely different. At eighty years old, I dressed as Eartha Kitt and mimed Santa Baby to the husband of one of the leaders who was dressed as Santa Claus. By the time we got to the end of the song, everyone was laughing and singing along. We had the group participating and having fun and it really broke the ice.
—Pat Stubbs, national secretary for the Volunteer Outreach Network; president of the West Virginia Community Educational Outreach Service

My elderly mother, Laurie, struggled with cancer for over three years. After several bouts of chemotherapy, she lost her hair as many do. The following doctor appointment she came armed with her Groucho Marx glasses, you know the ones with the big nose and big bushy eyebrows? She had her back to the door as the doctor entered the room. As he walked in, he routinely asked her how she was feeling from the chemotherapy treatments, as he looked down at her chart. She quickly turned around and surprised him by responding, "Well doc, I have lost all of my hair, but at least I still have my eyebrows!" We all started smiling and laughing. My mother was always trying to keep herself and those around her cheered up. She especially loved to make her oncologist laugh. She knew he had a tough job. My mom and I both believed her positive outlook and wonderful sense of humor helped her survive and thrive as well as she did during the course of her illness.
—Cynthia Keller, MA, mental health counselor

In creative problem solving, we often begin to solve a real problem by practicing on a mock problem such as "how to get an electric eel out of your toilet" or "how to get a hippo out of your bathtub." This

playful experience gets the creative juices flowing and places the real problem in a more productive perspective.
—Stavros Michailidis

3) What are the contents of your "bag of tricks" that you draw from to lift people's spirits?

A sense of ridiculousness, altruism, compassion, active listening skills, funny stories from my youth and a love to see others around me smile.
—David Smith, performing arts director, Robert M. Cooper Leadership Center

Smiles, impromptu thoughts, silly jokes, wacky behavior, the unexpected, silly songs, silly answers.
—Todd Moore and Janet Moore

A set of really bad jokes and a smile!
—Crystal Emerick, marketing and PR consultant

I try to make a personal connection with people. Getting to know somebody can cause the biggest smile of them all.
—Rocco Richard, recreation program supervisor, Chatham County Parks and Recreation

Utilizing what I know about someone and the things they enjoy, or just a funny picture!
—Claire Rutan

I like to know my audience before I even open my bag-o-tricks. There's nothing worse than using a type of humor that is not welcomed. This is where social awareness comes in. Social awareness, in my opinion, only works when you are able to understand your audience's "values." Values are at the core of humor. If they like "potty humor," a classic farting sound will put a smile on their face. But if your audience has more conservative values, they might need a small

dose of kindergarten or "punny" humor, something that won't make them uncomfortable. This is why some of the best jokes are told in private. We're prescribing the humor to just one person. My bag of tricks is vast but I never want to open a humor door unless I know I will be welcomed in. The other part of my bag of tricks that I rely on heavily is comedic timing. Comedic timing is nothing more than the ability to deliver a joke or punch line with a certain tempo that enhances the joke. I learned from the best. When I was younger and other kids were listening to music, I would listen to the greats: Bill Cosby, Eddie Murphy, Richard Pryor, Robin Williams, Steven Wright, Mitch Hedberg, and George Carlin. They all mastered comedic timing and did it in their own unique way. Because I listened to them on my Walkman (so my parents couldn't hear them) and didn't have the opportunity to see them perform, I tuned into their comedic timing. Today this allows me to see a moment for prescribing humor well before it arrives. Lastly, I rely on physical humor. For some reason I have a hard time memorizing jokes, but facial expressions that make people laugh have always come naturally. Acting or speaking like someone or something is a simple form of humor that is fun for the young and old.
—Pronto Parenteau

I just recall things from growing up. I come from a family of performers, musicians, and vaudeville, and I draw on family stories or memories. And I just use my own experiences through life. I also use myself a lot. For example, in the Red Hat society, I am known as "the girl with the big hat." I have this very large, oversized red hat with feathers. If I go somewhere, even men will comment, "Now that's a hat!"
—Pat Stubbs, national secretary for the Volunteer Outreach Network; president of the West Virginia Community Educational Outreach Service

Tell jokes, I'm "on" in conversation and use general conversation in a humorous way. I'll give off the wall answers to break the ice.
—Grit Thomas

Find the humor in everything, every situation and having the ability to laugh at myself.
—Patti Brown

I am more reminded of a specific trick that a friend of mine employs. At the most awkward, tense moment he gives someone a hug. This drops their guard, gets people enjoying themselves and creates positive motion.
—Stavros Michailidis

4) Sometimes humor therapy is an interaction between two people. Give an example of an interaction in which the conversation was therapeutic or uplifting.

Friend: I feel down today.
Me: I was just about to comment on your appearance.
Friend: What do you mean?
Me: What's the difference between a bucket of beautiful roses and you?
Friend: What?
Me: The bucket.
—David Smith, performing arts director, Robert M. Cooper Leadership Center

People like to feel they are understood. Giving someone permission and acceptance to feel whatever they feel can be a great relief. Sometimes a good listener is all you need to be. A great sense of humor helps you to be a good listener.
—Todd Moore and Janet Moore

Recently, a friend lost a job after four years of having no life or laughter due to work. Over a few glasses of wine, we joked about what was being left behind and savored what was to come for this friend. The lighthearted conversation and laughter left this person feeling optimistic.
—Crystal Emerick, marketing and PR consultant

My most memorable times that have been humorous and therapeutic have been when I'm spending time one on one with someone that has a similar sense of humor. My wife and my closest friends all have a similar sense of humor and that for me is very therapeutic—nothing is off limits! You name the type of humor and we've prescribed it for each other with positive results. The most therapeutic moments have been when I'm taking myself too seriously and a friend will use humor to break me out of the slump, similar to what I like to do with a camper that's having a bad day.
—Pronto Parenteau

My mother always had an answer. When I would get home after a frustrating day, she would say, "Why don't you eat? Things look better after you eat." Here is the rest of the story: if my answer was "I already ate!!!" then she would reply "Why don't you take a nap? Things look better after a nap ..."
—Maria Ferris, MD, PhD, MPH

Just respond with humor. Like when I had a surgeon with terrible bedside manner—almost creepy—and I couldn't have that. That's serious enough without laughing about it.
—Grit Thomas

My therapy dog Skittles and I were visiting a nursing home near my community recently, a place we frequent whenever we can. Several of the residents have become accustomed to seeing my toy poodle trotting through the halls, me on the side, and the activity director on the other as we go room to room. On this particular day, Miss Myrna (not her real name) rode up beside us in her wheelchair in the hallway, waiting to pet Skittles. I lifted the little seven-pound bundle and placed it in her lap. Miss Myrna's eighty-year-old eyes sparkled and she grinned with complete delight. Then Miss Myrna wrapped Skittles in a baby blanket as she petted her, telling me how much she loves dogs and misses having her own. Before I could reply, the wheelchair sped off (as much as a wheelchair powered by an elderly lady can speed off) with Skittles, still wrapped in the blanket! The activity director looked at me

with hilarious surprise. We both started laughing and following along behind, as Skittles and Miss Myrna went on a joy ride.
—Gina Farago, author

An overview between my brother and his girlfriend:

(Brother is driving a car; girlfriend is in the passenger seat. She is slightly annoyed at him for some reason. They pass by a church as the bride and groom are exiting.)

Brother: Look, a wedding.
Girlfriend: Aww, look at the bride, she's so pretty.
Brother: You know, I don't get weddings. It's just a made-up institution that blah, blah, blah …
Girlfriend: (angry) You're so insensitive sometimes!
Brother: What … what do you have against weddings?
(They both laugh together.)
—Stavros Michailidis

5) Sometimes humor therapy is self-prescribed. What do you do to enhance your own sense of humor and state of being?

Listen to children and remind myself what innocent humor sounds like before it matures into negative humor. I also laugh out loud (when I'm alone) just to remind myself how great it feels. I don't need funny visuals or jokes to do this. Weird, but man it feels great!
—David Smith, performing arts director, Robert M. Cooper Leadership Center

Thinking about things I do/have done to put smiles on kids' of all ages faces.
—Todd Moore and Janet Moore

I laugh at myself! Often it's my own mix-ups or goofiness that gives me the best joy, which—as my husband says—is odd.
—Crystal Emerick, marketing and PR consultant

Well I try to find something every day that will make me laugh. Most of the time it's a funny picture or video online. I print out my favorites and post them all around my desk. I also try to do silly things to make others laugh. Making someone else laugh brings me out of a funk.
—Rocco Richard, recreation program supervisor, Chatham County Parks and Recreation

Look at the positive side of things; there always is one!
—Claire Rutan

When I am particularly down or having a bad day, my husband asks me, "Is it a *Shrek* night?" No matter how bad a day I've had or how blue I am, watching *Shrek* will cheer me (or anyone) up. You can't watch the movie without laughing. I frequently quote Donkey: "I just know before this is over, I'm gonna need a whole lot of serious therapy. Look at my eye twitching." Another quote is "I'm a donkey on edge!" I have a little stuffed donkey in my office that I perch on the edge of things.
—Suzanne Williams-McAuliffe

I think of the fun and good times. I think of when I was working with David Mann and the silliness we all had together, the whole group. I think of the good things that make me smile or laugh.
—Pat Stubbs, national secretary for the Volunteer Outreach Network; president of the West Virginia Community Educational Outreach Service

I collect jokes, play with my cats, and approach situations with a light air.
—Grit Thomas

Take nothing seriously!
—Patti Brown

I try to stay aware of when I'm taking myself too seriously, and then I'll comment about myself. *Look at the silly human, he tries so hard. What does he really want? To be happy.* So then be happy, silly.
—Stavros Michailidis

6) Original thoughts, quotes, ideas about humor—anything that is truly original and personally yours.

When I was a kid I always wanted to do stand-up comedy. I was really shy but for some reason when I could get on a roll with jokes and make people laugh, all of those insecurities went away. For years I thought the funniest jokes were the ones that were made at someone else's expense; at least that is what seemed to work for all of the famous comics I saw on television. That strategy would get me a good laugh but I always felt bad about it. Two lessons I've learned being a camp director is that humor isn't always about jokes, and making people feel bad just isn't funny. Making other people laugh by pointing out the ridiculous and not being afraid to be silly is far more rewarding. A "good sense of humor" is not something you are born with but rather a way of viewing the world. The funniest and most fun people are able to find humor everywhere they go and are happier and healthier for it.
—Elaine Brinkley, Executive Director, Camp Fire Georgia

Laughing with friends is as good as eating fried gizzards because you want to.
—David Smith, Performing Arts Director, Robert M. Cooper Leadership Center

Sometimes you just have to sit and watch a squirrel.
—Daniel Hammond

Humor is a unique thing. Different people accept different types of humor and sometimes you have to get to know the person before you can really inject what is needed into the situation. *Smile, smile, smile!* And wiggle your ears!
—Todd Moore and Janet Moore

How often do I wish a humor box existed ... something you could preserve and open when you need a laugh or to smile. However, when I look around the world, that box of smiles actually does exist. For each of us, it's different but it can be a beautiful bird, lighthearted '50s song, a sweet-smelling flower or the smile of a loved one. The challenge is actually taking the time to recognize and embrace those daily joys.
—Crystal Emerick, marketing and PR consultant

There are times when you just gotta laugh ... because we don't want people to see the real emotions behind the laugh.
—Mary Treece, Child Protective Services worker

Smile! It makes life easier! Plus it gives you less wrinkles!
—Claire Rutan

Growing up I learned very quickly that if I wasn't going to be tall, dark and handsome, I'd better be funny! The way to a woman's heart has been and always will be *food* (just kidding) ... it's humor. One of the first things we say we want in a partner is someone that can make me laugh. This is because we all want to laugh and have someone to laugh with. That's why I believe humor is therapeutic.
—Pronto Parenteau

My humor feels like Cheerwine, goes down smooth but jolts you with energy!
—Stew Harsant

Is there such a thing as reverse humor therapy? At the hospital I'm around patients a lot so when I meet someone who tries to be humorous with me I spend extra time with them and go along with it. That makes them feel good knowing they are making me laugh ... or that I'm willing to hang around to listen and talk. I guess I do that with everyone I work with too. It might not be that funny but I go along with it most of the time so they keep a smile.
—Joe Dennis

We need more humor therapy in the world!
—Pat Stubbs, national secretary for the Volunteer Outreach Network; president of the West Virginia Community Educational Outreach Service

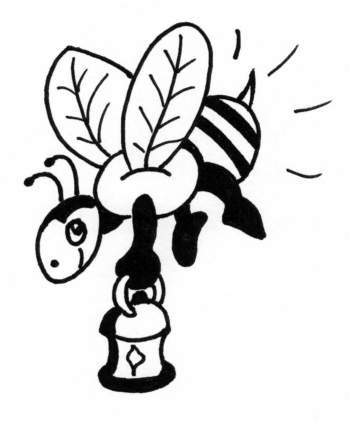

If you don't laugh like you do at home … you should be.

CHAPTER 6

EXTRA TOOLS FOR YOUR DOCTOR'S BAG

This last chapter is filled with a variety of items to use at will. Different therapy situations call for different humor tools. Somewhere in this chapter you will find just the right humor therapy pun, poem, sight gag, or song that matches perfectly to someone you care for. Familiarize yourself with the humor items, and please remember, use only what you need and no more. Don't overdo it with one laugh after another. Use the precise amount of humor starters that will lift up others and brighten their day, and then quickly connect with their hearts. Your participation and involvement will heal in ways you never imagined. Now get out there and look for stressed out friends, miserable coworkers in the next cubicle, or family members going through hard times. Your smile is the starting point, and the humor you prescribe is waiting inside your imaginary doctor's bag. While you are doing all of this superhero work, keep it intentional and *smile for others*.

SIGHT GAGS

Phone attached to a boomerang: "Does your phone have *call return*?"
Baby bibs sewed to overalls: "Like my *bib overalls*?"
Photo of a hand in a baggie: "I bought my wife a new *handbag*."
Tape measure: "Don't worry, this won't take *long*."
Toy rabbit with a small piece of netting: "Need a *hair net*?"
Stuffed toy seal: "I named my pet *seal Easter*."
Stick with plastic lips attached: "Anyone lose their *lip stick*?"
Wear two hats: "Okay, let's *recap*."
Doorknob: "Wanna see something to *adore*?"

CONVERSATION TOOLS

I laughed out loud last week when I _____.

I laugh to myself every time I _____.

It was not that funny at the time, but now I laugh when I think of_____.

My favorite cartoon is still_____.

I amuse myself when _____.

As a child, I remember laughing at _____.

At work, I think it's funny when _____.

It may sound childish, but I laugh at _____.

In general, people are just silly when they _____.

The funniest outfit I ever wore was _____.

Life is like a bucket of snails. Here's why_____.

Life is funny. Let me give you an example: _____.

The funniest person I personally know is _____. Here's why.

The funniest thing I ever saw an animal do was _____.

My sense of humor is like a _____.

Walk into any supermarket and I see humor in the _____ aisles. Here's why.

The hardest and loudest laugh I ever experienced was the time _____.

Here are a few out-of-the-blue conversational questions that might cause a grin or smile:

What's it like to be you?

Is it fun to be like that?

Is it true that the word *screeched* is the longest one-syllable word in the dictionary?

Can you repeat that with a little more zest?

What do you have to say for yourself?

What is the weirdest thing you have ever eaten?

For more in-depth responses (and subsequent laughs), the following are a few mild debate topics that inspire silliness!

What do you do to insure that a hot dog is spaced equally between the ends of the bun? And if it is placed closer to one of the ends, how do you deal with the last bite of only mustard, slaw, and other ingredients?

Which is better: to use a straw to taste the bottom of the glass of lukewarm undiluted cola, or not use a straw and sip from the top of the glass to taste the ice-cold diluted drink?

Pizza bones: do you eat the crust after eating the rest of the slice, save it for dipping, or toss aside to be trashed?

Why is it said that you're never too old to learn but you can't teach an old dog new tricks?

Why is the pen mightier than the sword, but actions speak louder than words?

How come the devil is in the details, but one should not sweat the small stuff?

Why do birds of a feather flock together, but opposites attract?

How come the clothes make the man, but you should not judge a book by its cover?

How come haste makes waste, but you should make hay while the sun shines?

Which is better ___or___? Would you rather ___or___? (Add your own to complete)

Think of any mild debate that promotes a positive discussion of silly options, funny decisions, and/or humorous thinking.

Ask someone to explain or simply discuss any of the following tidbits:
Everyone's going to the pier. Is that peer pressure?

Is there anything you don't know? I don't know.

I tried that positive thinking stuff. I knew it wouldn't work and sure enough, it didn't.

Thirty divided by one half is sixty (not fifteen). Thirty divided by two is fifteen.

What was the president's name in 1990? The answer is always the current president; his name never changed.

How far can you run into the woods? The answer is only half way because after the mid-point you are running out of the woods.

How long is a piece of string? The answer is twice the length of one of its ends to the middle of the string.

If I run down a moving escalator am I not traveling into the future?

While gazing into a mirror you are actually looking at yourself twice the distance from the mirror to your face.

How can you see yourself sneezing if your eyes always close during the sneeze?

Why is saliva disgusting outside your mouth but just fine inside your mouth?

How old would you be if you didn't know how old you were?

Where is your funny bone?

RECIPES

I've discovered that a simple dinner invite can raise the spirits of anyone. For someone feeling down, this can be an evening to forget about things and explore the senses. It can do wonders. The following recipes incorporated into a meal can bring on some serious funny conversations.

Recipe from Cecelia Hart-Hodges
CeCe has a strategy for adding zest to a friend who is feeling low in spirits. She invites him or her over for dinner and serves bacon-wrapped dates (with an almond next to the date). This isn't a very common appetizer and begs the question "Ever tried these?" followed by the comment "Well, everyone should have great dates in their lives." After explaining the recipe, how they are made, and how funny the supermarket clerk looks at you when you say you are looking for *dates*, a smile, even a small one will develop.

Recipe from Mack Dennis
"When I was a little kid I remember butchering day at my grandfather's farm. Mom and Dad would help with the butchering. They would cure the hams, make sausage, and can other parts. Mom even had use for the pig's tail. The end where it was cut off had a lot of fat on it. She would use the whole tail to grease the griddle when she made pancakes. When it came to butchering cows, the tongue was a special treat. Here's how to cook it."

Delightful Beef Tongue
1 beef tongue with blood and slobber washed off
1 medium onion
1 large garlic clove
salt and pepper to taste

Place tongue in stew pot with enough water to cover. Add onion, garlic, salt, and pepper. Cover and simmer for 2 1/2 hours. When done, remove the tongue to cutting board. Then remove the white skin from the tongue. Slice the tongue into 1/2-inch slices. Can be used in sandwiches or free style with veggies. This is not for wimps. However, it is very tasty with melted Swiss cheese over it and a slice of mild onion. Will put hair on your chest.

Recipe from David Smith

In grade school our math teacher told the class how to cook worms. No, this is not the famous Halloween recipe that uses noodles or gummy worms placed in a cup of chocolate pudding and crushed Oreo cookies. This one was told in such detail and description that even today, I believe it!

Wonderful Fried Worms

1 handful of live red wigglers or night crawlers
1 shoebox of flour or cornmeal
deep fryer

Place the worms into the shoebox filled with flour or cornmeal for a week or so. Watch for the worms to fade and turn pale. As they eat and tunnel through the flour they process out the gritty dirt and fill up with the smooth eatable flour. Keep in shoebox until worm poop is light in color. Then take worms out and throw in deep fryer. Cook until they curl up and are lightly browned.
Salt and pepper to taste.

Recipe from my dad

I have on occasion taken purple pickled eggs to a friend's house to lighten the mood. With all seriousness involved, I have a great recipe that was created by my father that includes vinegar, pickled beet juice, bay leaves, pickling spices, and a secret ingredient that I will never give up. After three weeks in a jar stored in the cupboard, the purple color bleeds halfway into each egg. Once sliced in half, they are beautiful to look at as well as eat! Humor is easy to share when the topic of discussion is pickled eggs, the variations of how to make them, plus the puzzled looks of "Why?"

PUNS

I particularly like puns because they cast a broad net to all encountered. Hidden in a professional conversation, I can slip in a profession-related pun that is not third-grade level. Plus, I can pull out the silliest pun to prompt a smile on a preschooler. In fact, what I call *snowball jokes* can open the door for anyone to participate. They are called this because they start small and grow as others get into them. These jokes are quick humor bits that anyone can build upon. I'm pleasantly pleased when I tell one or two snowball jokes only to see them return within a few minutes. People are usually excited to have the opportunity to share something that they think they come up with all on their own.

Examples include:

I always wanted to be a violin player, but I was too "high strung."
I always wanted to be a banker, but then I lost "interest."
I always wanted to be in a profession that works on beds, but that job has not been "made up" yet.
I always wanted to be a teacher, but I had no "class."
I always wanted to be a plumber, but that was just a "pipe dream."

After only a couple of these, others will propose one. The secret is that practically every profession has a pun hidden in its description. You just have to seek it out. Dentists stick to the drill, accountants know what counts, physicists care about what matters, roof repairs are over my head, and so on.

More puns:

My dentist gets way too personal. He's always asking me about my fillings.
My entire family thinks I'm indecisive. I'm not so sure about that.

An artist was arrested for a holdup. Cops say that details are sketchy.

Working in a bakery is great if you knead the dough.

Port-a-potties at the crime prevention fair were all stolen. Police trainees have nothing to go on.

My doctor told me that I had a bladder infection by saying "urine trouble."

Have you heard about the book titled *Understanding Anti-Gravity*? You won't be able to put it down.

A bottle of Windex tried to catch some fog, but he mist.

Thief damage leaves large hole in the side of lingerie store wall. Police are looking into it.

POEMS/SONGS

Sometimes a poem can remind you of how blissful it was to be a playful youth. Simply reading or singing the following can spark conversations with a smile.

Feeling Young

Walk on down my street and chase a few pebbles
And lose all conception of time
We'll play make-believe, like airplanes and gliders
And sitting on the ground would be a crime
Well you know and I know that feeling young just begun today

So climb an ole oak tree and swing on its branches
And see how dirty we can get
Then I'll wear my dad's coat and you wear some makeup
And we'll pretend we just met
Well you know and I know that feeling young just begun today

You be the princess and I'll rule the kingdom
We'll laugh at each other till we hurt
We'll live in a castle where all is forgotten
It's that much fun in the dirt
Well you know and I know that feeling young just begun today

Drive on down your street and chase a few dollars
And keep your conception of time
You play reality with grown-ups and big kids
And silly games are a crime
Well you know and I know that feeling young just begun today

Walk on down my street and chase a few pebbles
And lose all conception of time
We'll play make-believe the way that we want to
And trying to act big would be a crime
Well you know and I know that feeling young just begun today

Well maybe this song is intended for children
Laughing and singing in the sun
Or maybe this song is intended for grown-ups
Laughing but missing all the fun

This Matt Dillon sing-along was written to replace the traditional "Dem Bones" campfire song. It's a blend of the Adam and Eve story and the *Gunsmoke* TV series.

Matt Dillon
The Lord decided to make a little town
He took a little water and took a little ground
He stirred that ground round and round
And made Dodge City without another sound
Well out of that mud and dirt and clay
He made Matt Dillon, Doc, and Festus Ray
But ole Matt Dillon was lonesome blue
And the Lord didn't know just what to do
So he took a rib from ole Matt's side
And made Miss Kitty to be his bride
Well buckles and broncos and all that such
But from that saloon thou dare not touch
Cause around that saloon ole Satan slunk
And that ole devil gets everyone drunk
Here comes the devil, all blood and flesh
(Kitty) "Matt, Matt Dillon, I think he's gettin' fresh
(Devil) "Kitty, my liquor tastes mighty fine
Take a little sip, the Lord won't mind"
So she took a little sip and then a little drink

Forty drinks later, Kitty couldn't think
Next day later, the Lord came round
Spied those bottles and shot glasses on the ground
(Lord) "*Mat, Matt Dillon, where art thou?*"
(Mat) "Here I am Lord just riding my cow."
(Lord) "*Well, Matt Dillon, who drank up my city?*"
(Mat) "I don't know Lord, it must have been Kitty."
(Lord) "*Well, Matt Dillon, you must leave my town.*
Take your ole cow and don't hang around."
So Matt took his ride and then he took his time
That's why drinking is still a dirty crime
So now Matt Dillon is living on a farm
Just milking his cow and doing no harm
But his cow keeps kicking him over the fence
Cause he tries to milk his cow with a monkey wrench
Now don't forget Doc, he's old as a rock
Never had trouble until he swallowed his clock
Now he's lost all zest and zime
Just sits in the back, trying to pass time
And Ole Festus Ray bought a mathematical dog
Broke his little paw on a hollow log
But the dog still thinks that counting is fun
Cause he puts down three and carries one
Well liquor is quicker and wine is fine
But it's all a bunch of trouble, if the advice were mine
So have a big party and invite me to it
But keep your ole liquor cause I ain't gonna do it

This next song was written to sing around the 4-H campfires. I got
the idea from the camp song called "Great Big Gobs of Greasy Grimy
Gopher Guts" which is just as disgusting. My "Booger Song" took on a
life of its own and is still occasionally sung in southern West Virginia
when adults allow it.

"Booger Song"

Picking boogers on a sunny day
Stick your finger up all the way
Shake it around and let it play
Pull it out and say "Lunch today"

Picking boogers on a moony night
Pull the snot out with all your might
Do it and chew it but do it right
Cause every booger's got a big delight

Picking boogers was Mabel and I
We picked a whole handful and that's no lie
A slimy long and green one was what I just found
But before I got to keep it, Mabel gobbled it down

Picking boogers on a sunny day
Stick your finger up all the way
Shake it around and let it play
Pull it out and say "Lunch today"

I pick so many boogers I hide them everywhere
I poke them in my pocket and I rub them in my hair
I got some in the kitchen and even in the hall
When I get them on my finger I wipe them on the wall

It's oozing on my finger so lick it if you dare
But don't let Daddy catch you hiding them under his chair
I got them in the bedroom and even in the den
When I get them on my finger I flip them off again

Picking boogers on a sunny day
Stick your finger up all the way
Shake it around and let it play
Pull it out and say "Lunch today"

STORIES

Humor stories from our past can bring smiles to family members during holiday get-togethers and reunions. They promote family traditions and the art of generational oral histories. Everybody has these. What are yours? Do you share them?

Vacation story from Helen Hardman
I just got back from Florida from a three-week vacation with Terry. We laughed from Wytheville, Virginia, to Horner, West Virginia, because we watched two guys trying to get kerosene into a container. When the one guy, Bubba #1, finally put the kerosene can into the back of the truck, the other guy, Bubba # 2, got in on the passenger side. When Bubba #1 tried to open the driver side truck door with a hard jolt, the entire door fell off. He just scratched his head and Bubba # 2 just sat in the front seat smiling. Well Terry and I both scrambled for our cameras as we laughed and wiped tears. Well Bubba #1 jumped in the back of the truck and got a broom and used it as a wedge and tried to pry the door back on. Terry was going to go to his rescue but he couldn't stop laughing. Bubba # 2 sat calmly by just watching! When he got the door wedged up on one bottom hinge, it wouldn't close shut. He proceeded to jump in the back of his pickup once again and got a sledgehammer and commenced to beating on the truck door to get it shut. All of a sudden, he noticed dents coming into play ... go figure that! Terry said, "Uh oh, what's he going to do next? Oh no, not the full body slam." Sure enough, he threw himself into the door and *voila*, it closed. Then he calmly picked up broom and hammer and threw them back into the truck, scratched his head and wondered how in the devil do I get in the truck now? So he did what every other Nascar fan and/or driver would do; he decided to jump into the window. Now that truck was parked on a slanting little embankment of concrete and his legs were pretty short at best. Well, he gave a thrust and one leg went over the windowsill and then his head and alas ... he was hung! Well Bubba #2, decided to help out

his friend finally. He gave a big old pull and Bubba #1 torpedoed into the truck cab right across the seat and landed into his companion's midsection with a *thud*. He was backward and looking toward the bed of the truck instead of the steering wheel. Well, as I cried tears of laughter and joy, the two large men tried to wiggle around then finally got Bubba #1 under the steering wheel and they headed out! As I laughed more and more, they pulled onto I-77 and as they went around the curve to go on the highway ... you guessed it, the door popped open. Terry and I finally stopped laughing and headed in the opposite direction on the highway, praying for their safety and shaking our heads.

High school story from Joe Dennis

A girl that sat in front of me in class had long black hair. I asked her for one of her hairs. She plucked it out for me. I caught a fly by trapping it against the classroom window with my hand. My friend, who sat next to me, then held it down on the desk while I looped the hair around its neck. I took a piece of tape and taped the end of the hair to the desk. My friend let the fly go and it looked like it was on a leash tethered to the desk. It was flying around and not going anywhere pulling on the hair. It was great! At my class reunion, that girl was there and that's the first I've seen her since high school. She told that story of the fly and said that was one of her favorite memories.

Grade school story from David Smith

I was focused on cutting out a paper puppet from a children's magazine. The pieces were detailed so it took the better part of arts class. Midway through my effort, Mrs. Wills, my teacher, looked over my shoulder and commented loud enough for the entire class to hear, "David, it seems like every time you start a hard project, you see it through to the end." I actually laughed out loud. In my mind, her comment was not true. How silly of her. I just wanted this one paper puppet really bad and was really focused on it. But, as soon as she spoke, I looked at the rest of the classroom and noticed that all the other students were looking at me and believing her praise. At that moment, her words become real and the trait of finishing things I start stuck with me for a lifetime. Even after all these years, when I think of this story, I smile inside. It's true that thirty seconds of supporting someone's self-esteem can change the person's life forever.

ODDS AND ENDS

Seven levels of laughter (you always have options)
I'm walking down the street and I see someone slip on a banana peel without harming himself.
After asking "You okay?" what do you do?

1) I barely smile.
2) I grin boldly.
3) I chuckle under my breath.
4) I laugh in a low tone.
5) I laugh "Ha!"
6) I burst out with a vociferous "Ha Ha!"
7) I throw my head back, my face turns red, my entire body rocks, I slap my leg, I drop to the ground laughing loudly, and I check with others around me and ask "Did you see that?"

Unfinished proverbs
Examples: No sense crying over spilled *Visine*. A bird in the hand is worth *two at KFC*.
A fool and his money are_____.
A penny saved is a penny_____.
Actions speak louder than_____.
Blood is thicker than water but_____.
Curiosity killed the_____.
Don't count your chickens before they_____.
Haste makes_____.
The bigger they are, the harder they_____.
You can't judge a book by its cover, but_____.

There are many ways to make a funny face:

the face one makes to prompt a baby to smile
the face one makes while winking one eye

the face one makes that requires the use of fingers
the face one makes while posing in the family picture
the face one makes that enhances a comic high-browed stare
the face one makes that accompanies a rolling of the eyes;.
the face one makes to demonstrate a puzzled look
the face that accompanies the look of *aw shucks*
the face one makes when using a wide-open mouth
the face one makes that demonstrates *sourness*
the face one makes to display the ability to wiggle one's nose or ears
the face one makes when pretending to be mad but the look is overshadowed by a grin
the face one makes when expressing the mood of romance
the face one makes when one encounters a new toy
the face one makes to mirror someone else up close to get him or her to grin
the face one makes when they are imitating fish
the face one makes while touching her tongue to her nose
the face one makes when she realizes that this went on a bit too long
the face one makes at knowing that I lost half the readers in the first ten faces

Now make a funny face right now; nobody is watching. You'll feel like an expert!

TWENTY THINGS TO TRY

1) Wear a tie-dyed shirt to a gathering, and spray your hair with one of those Halloween-colored hair sprays. Wear an outfit with bright colors, or wear a neon hat to complete the effect. Walk up to folks, and ask, "Guess what happened to me?" You might have a prepared punch line up your sleeve, but don't share it yet. Wait for their responses. They then have the opportunity to state a funny comment that captures your silly look. They also get the first chance to complete the humor moment right in front of a ready-made audience while you remain the willing target. If they are hesitant or suggest no comments at all, then offer up something like "Someone on the way in said I looked like I just wrestled a clown. What do you think?" You now have opened the door for short-term humor and one-liners with minimum involvement. You might hear comments such as:

   You look like you slept with a box of crayons under your pillow.
   You look like you just crawled out of the world's largest bag of Skittles.
   You look like you just finished your first cosmetology class.
   You look like you have been eating too many jelly beans.

   Whatever the comment, smile, and let them know you did this for them. They will be talking about it for years.

2) Ask friends to give silly descriptors to common items—for example, "What is a spoon best used for?" Answers might include something like

   a snow sled for mice;
   an alien eye patch;
   a big-toe protector; or
   a circus fun mirror for turtles.

3) Next time a relative has to stay in the hospital for a week or so, buy a dozen get-well cards that are all the same. Mail them to family members across the country. Tell them to send them back to the relative in the hospital within the next few days. As the first one arrives, it will be cute, but as the rest of them are delivered, the patient will quickly know that it was all planned in advance. Humor will be in the discussions for years about how the family planned together to pull this off. Isn't it super nice when others put effort into your feeling better?

4) While sitting in a public park or mall, look for

anything plaid;
things that are fuzzy;
items that are cartoon shaped;
people who are celebrity look-alikes;
things that are outright funny; or
anything that appears incongruent.

5) Make yourself a name-tag sticker with *I Y Q* written on it. When someone asks what it means, tell him or her to say the letters out loud. After he or she does this, respond with "I wike you too."

6) In a group setting or gathering, divide the group into three imaginary sections to create a three dimensional sneeze. Give the first section the word "Hishy," and have them repeat it back to you out loud. The second section gets the word "Hooshy," and the third gets "Hashy." Have them all say their words together at the same time. Finish with your response of "Gesundheit."

7) Look at a digital clock sideways (tilt your head 90 degrees to the left), and view sketch faces at any time of day. The hour number displays the eyebrows and top of the head, the colon displays the eyes, and the minutes display everything else on a face (cheeks, mustache, mouth, beard, chin, and so forth).

8) While stressed-out customers wait in line at a grocery store, add humor to the moment by reading out loud the headlines of those silly gossip-news magazines. Humor just might rub off onto others.

9) Next time you are on an elevator, share this joke with others:

Did you know that if Ella Fitzgerald married Darth Vader, she would be Ella Vader?

10) If you look at anything in this world with squinted eyes, you can see whatever you creatively want to.

11) Look through a square piece of plexiglass while gazing at clouds. Use a dry-erase marker to outline the things you see while sharing with others.

12) Hand a folded piece of paper to someone you know, and in a low tone, say, "This is for you. Please open it later." When he or she does open it, the only thing written is the letter *U*.

13) Prior to falling asleep at night, think about funny moments of your life. Your dreams will be more lighthearted.

14) Lick your own finger, and stick it in your ear. Laugh out loud. This simply reinforces the fact that you still have a sense of ridiculousness. Plus it gives you a chance to remove dry flakes from your ears.

15) Have a conversation with your spouse, and pretend that you are still in high school. Remember how to flirt, wink, and write silly love poems.

16) When in a stressful interaction with a colleague or supervisor, I use thought exaggerations like imagining the person's head changing shape or enlarging as he talks on and on. I imagine his head

spinning completely around when he is being circumloquacious. Hey, it's a real word. It's when someone talks in circles. Didn't I use this word earlier in this book?

17) At a fast-food restaurant, unfold a paper napkin, and cover your entire face with it. Ask, "Want to see something you have never seen before?" After getting everyone's attention, poke your tongue through the paper napkin, and wiggle it.

18) Next time you see an empty desk in a lobby, sit behind it, and set up a Free Advice sign.

19) For group discussion fun, obtain two copies of a DVD cartoon. Play the same DVD in two different rooms. One room gets only the sound while the other room gets only the picture. Come together, and discuss what was funny.

20) Start a laughter meet-up group, or plan weekly friendship get-togethers. Use the following as the group's agenda or vision statement. This group is for everyone who wants to explore a variety of ways of promoting positive, uplifting humor. Along the way, we will pursue ways to prescribe humor to others who may be in need of a good laugh.
Activities and outings may include watching funny movies, reviewing humor books, going out to lunch just to share clean jokes, visiting senior citizen homes or hospitals, researching ways to present humor better, learning a few humor tricks to entertain the family during holiday gatherings, and looking at humor styles. Please remember that Debbie Downers, Negative Nancys, and Mean Matthews might want to seek out other groups that better fit what they are looking for. The intent here is to share positive, uplifting ideas and plan fun outings. Together we will learn how to *smile for others*.
Disclaimer ... At no time will we as members share humor or jokes that offend, degrade, or stereotype others. Political, religious, or racial humor is generally not acceptable.

If there is one concept from this book to remember, let it be this. Everyone carries with him or her an imaginary doctor's bag filled with fun, hope, and humor tools. Share and prescribe to those in need. Seek them out as they are counting on you. Thanks again for taking the time to learn how to *smile for others*.

The End ... or is it?

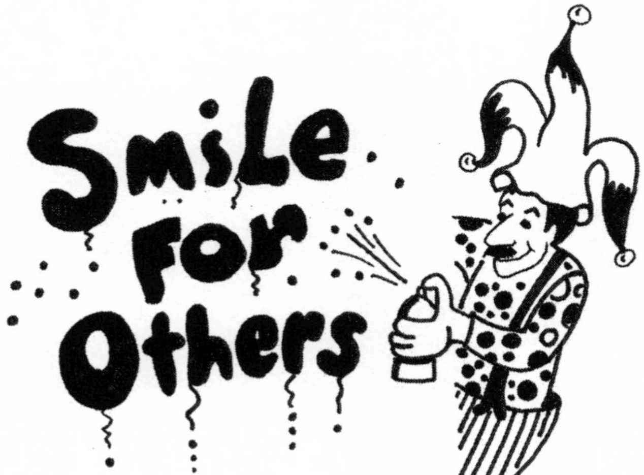
Smile For Others

Made in the USA
Middletown, DE
30 July 2018